LIFE IN THE HOUSE OF CARDS
(Or Parenting a Child with Mental Illness)
Irene Abramovich, M.D., Ph.D.

LIFE IN THE HOUSE OF CARDS
(Or Parenting a Child with Mental Illness)
Irene Abramovich, M.D., Ph.D.

iUniverse, Inc.
Bloomington

iUniverse books may be ordered through booksellers or by contacting:

iUniverse
1663 Liberty Drive
Bloomington, IN 47403
www.iuniverse.com
1-800-Authors (1-800-288-4677)

ISBN: 978-1-4620-7204-0 (sc)
ISBN: 978-1-4620-7206-4 (hc)
ISBN: 978-1-4620-7205-7 (ebk)
Printed in the United States of America
iUniverse rev. date: 12/28/2011

ACKNOWLEDGMENTS

My first thanks are to Mrs. L. Anderson, Mrs. L. Hamilton, Mrs. C. Lawson, Mrs. B. Mertz, Mrs. L. Mariebelle, and T. Strom: Without your contribution writing this book would not be possible.

Mrs. L. Anderson and Mrs. T. Strom: your encouragement, feedback, sharing the invaluable knowledge and experience were an ongoing inspiration.

My family: my most severe critics and first readers.

Sergei and Nikita Prokhorov: you created the unique cover and graphic design, capturing the spirit and the soul of this book I could only dream of.

Jorge Sanchez and K.B: you bravely opened the door to the world we would never know about.

Diane Valentine: my forever partner in our travel into the depth of education and psychology, making the most complicated issues easy to understand.

To R. and S.
With love and gratitude.

Juvela Obi

You lean on me
And I lean on you
Like a house of cards
We stand

Without the one
The other would fall
So like a house of cards
We stand

Alone I don't have the strength
To bear this weight
And neither alone has the base
To stand up straight

But if we lean on each other
We triple our strength
And if we lean on each other
Two bases are one

I'll share my weight
And you'll share yours
And together
We'll make each other strong

Table Of Contents

Preface

Dear Reader, this book isn't a scientific research, or a navigation guide in a stormy ocean of child psychiatry. Neither is it a "cookbook" with recipes and suggestions on how to manage a child with a mental illness. This book was born as a result of years of shared experience with the parents of young patients, struggling with the same questions, as they tread through the mental health medical community. This work is inspired by the parents; it is dedicated to the parents and is about the parents and their children with mental illness. Together, with shared family stories and psychiatric knowledge we try to answer some thorny and raw questions.

This story started more than ten years ago when a seven-year-old boy walked into my office holding his parents' hands. The gloomy expression of his little face was in a stark contrast to his upbeat parents' demeanor. The parents were accomplished professionals, who adored their only child and did not believe that something could possibly be wrong with him. They came to me yielding to the school request to see a psychiatrist, as the school psychologist suggested, that little Evan had "school phobia," and the family needed to come up with "a behavioral plan." Indeed, Evan had always been an outgoing and sociable child, well liked by his peers and adults, and a stellar student. A couple of months prior to our meeting, he refused to go to school, all of a sudden. Evan cried every morning and even attempted to hide in the closet where he believed he could not be found. Nobody could understand this turn in his behavior: he still performed very well academically and remained popular at school. I was left alone with Evan; he was looking down sitting on the chair almost motionlessly. When I asked why he did not want to go to school, he said in a hardly audible voice: "Because the monsters are telling me not to," and tears rolled down his cheeks. I started asking him more questions about those monsters, how he heard them, and what they looked like. Upon realizing that his revelation did not at all surprise me, Evan looked up at me for the first time and the words started pouring out of him. As it turned out, nobody had ever asked him the magic question "why". The adults around Evan, who truly cared about him, were asking if the teacher or other kids did not treat him well, if he was not feeling all right, if he found the academics difficult. He was afraid to reveal his secret thinking, that nobody would believe him.

He was a smart kid...Evan told me that he started hearing monsters' voices a couple of months ago. They were constantly telling him, that he would die, that his parents would die in a car accident when he is at school, that other children did not like him and only pretended being his friends. Evan's mood was sinking, as the monsters were telling him, that he would rather be dead than alive. As soon as the lights turned off, Evan would see the monsters flying into his room, leaning over his bed, whispering threats into his ears. He stopped sleeping. Evan seemed to be relieved, that he shared his secret with somebody, who obviously took it seriously. He even smiled for the first time, when I explained, that we were going to help him. Now it was his parents turn. Is there a good way to explain to the parents, that their child has no "school phobia," but instead suffers from a psychotic episode? If there is – I wish I knew it! The moment, when a scary, threatening diagnosis must be delivered to the parents, is painfully difficult for any physician. A split second separates a wholesome, happy life, with a bright future and hopes of raising a normal, healthy child, going to baseball games and band recitals, from a totally different world, filled with fears and uncertainty, visits to doctors, treatments, and side effects of medications at times as bad as the disease they treat. So, such moment of truth for Evan's parents came.

The news is released: the mother's expression changes from a pleasant smile, to an incredulous look, to an angry mask and at last to tears. The father's mouth turns into a white hard line. The "grief cycle" first described in such a succinct way by Dr. Elizabeth

Kubler-Ross, including sequential stages of denial, anger, bargaining, depression and acceptance, flashed before of my eyes. The parents were grieving the loss of a normal child. It was a shock, an unbelievable, impossible event, which could not have happened to their sweet little kid! On the other hand, the details they heard and the timing of the behavioral changes left little doubt, that it was anything but true. Still, I suggested getting a second opinion, which came later from a therapist. After sharing the secret with me, Evan felt comfortable talking about his monsters and voices. He repeated what he said to me to his therapist, working with him on a behavioral modification plan. The parents receive similar feedback for the second time and now they seek medical help. Part two of our conversation, not less difficult than the first one, is about helping Evan with medications. The parents go through a conventional array of questions about "natural" approach, counseling, and the possibility of "attention deficit", still not ready for the acceptance of the medical reality dawning on them...Many years have passed, and Evan has grown up into a fine young man, who had a painfully close encounter with mental illness and has become an expert in it. He went through trials of different medications, sometimes feeling "normal," and sometimes the disease consuming him. But through all his ordeals he remained smart and insightful, never letting his condition take over his personality, being as charming and successful academically as he had always been. His parents stood by him, meeting the disaster fearlessly, looking the monsters right into the eyes and conquering it with the love and knowledge they acquired through the years. They learned about medications and the disease more, than anybody would imagine, offering their support and wisdom to other parents new to this field.

Since then, hundreds of children, adolescents and their parents have walked into my office. Working as a consultant for a school district, I met with many families, where children were suffering from different psychiatric conditions. Some of the parents joined the troops fighting mental illness and some of them left my office (sometimes angrily) still not convinced, that childhood mental illnesses beside ADHD exist.

The most dramatic encounter I've had was with the family of one of my colleagues, an adult psychiatrist, who brought his twelve-year-old son after failing multiple previous treatments for "ADHD." This young man, Derek, did not hesitate to tell me about different voices he had been hearing for the last five years (approximately the length of time he was treated for the ADHD condition). He was bright and eloquent, describing the whole world of aliens intruding his mind, interfering with his thoughts and not allowing him to do any work at school. Derek's attention definitely was not good, but for a totally different reason. After one of many psychiatrists he was seeing put him on Prozac, Derek started feeling like a superman. He made a swing out of the rope, hanging it between two floors in his house and was riding it wildly, screaming with delight. Even after a fire brigade came with a ladder to take him off this makeshift swing and the ambulance had to inject him with sedatives, the father did not change his mind about "ADHD" origin of the problem. I met with Derek and his family soon after this episode. Derek told me that voices were louder after he took Prozac and encouraged him to make the swing and ride it. I convinced the parents to start Derek on a low dose of an anti-psychotic medication which dramatically improved his condition as well as the attention span, but his father remained angry and terminated Derek's treatment with me, because I refused to accept his diagnostic concept and disagreed that Derek just had a company of "imaginary friends" and a difficult to treat case of ADHD.

So, when a pediatric specialist, an allergist for example, would present the parents with a medical diagnosis of any kind, the parents would do their best to follow the medical recommendations to a tee. Time and again I found, that this principle does not apply to child psychiatry: the psychiatric diagnosis would cause anger and disbelief, prompting many parents to contest it. Why has child psychiatry become a "Cinderella" in medicine? And what are the historical roots of child psychiatry?

Chapter 1
What's in a Name (of Child Psychiatry)?

People always had to fight mental illnesses. In prehistoric times, a mental illness was believed to be inflicted by magic creatures invading the mind. Accordingly, shamans used spells and rituals in order to provide the exorcism to get rid of them. They also practiced some primitive surgery, drilling a hole into the skull, which would allow evil spirits to leave the head and free the sick man. Skulls with those holes dating back more than 10,000 years have been found in Neolithic Europe and South America. About 400 B.C., the Greek physician Hippocrates stated, that mental disorders were caused by an imbalance of four body fluids: blood, phlegm, yellow bile, and black bile.

In ancient Egypt mental illnesses were also believed to be magical or religious in nature, but still some attempts were made to approach it "medically." The first psychiatric text was written around 2nd century BC, explaining the causes of hysteria and mentioning the first psychiatric hospital. In the first mental institution they prescribed opium to induce visions, performed rituals or prayers to appease gods, and used sleep therapy, interpreting the dreams to discover the nature of the illness. The Egyptians paid a lot of attention to the health of the soul, presenting the first example of mental healthcare as a high priority.

The next step in understanding the nature of mental illnesses can be traced back to ancient Jews. In Judaism, the first monotheistic religion, mental problems were believed to be caused by a conflict in the relationship between the ill man and God. The illness was seen as possession by demons and a sin. The treatment accor-dingly was prayers, fasting, and self flagellation. On the other hand, mental health was essential and valued as the foundation for a healthy relationship with God.

Early Islam also focused on the understanding of mental health. Mentally ill were believed to be possessed by either good or bad spirits, and this is why the supernatural invasion of the brain was not always interpreted as bad or sinful. Such removal of the stigma from insanity as being "wrong" opened the door for a more scientific look at the causes and presentations of mental illness. A manuscript describing symptoms of mental illness and the treatments had been written in the 10th century. There was also a psychiatric ward in Baghdad hospital.

On the other hand, in Europe, mental illness was still perceived as a demonic possession. During the Medieval times, especially the Reformation, belief in the witchcraft and the wide persecution of witches spread throughout the Western Europe. People with mental illness were considered witches and burned or incarcerated. Drilling holes in the skull to release the presumed malevolent spirit inside remained a common procedure from prehistoric times through the 1800s. Various methods were undertaken on schizophrenic individuals in an effort to quell psychotic episodes. Dr. Benjamin Rush, an American physician, believed that all mental illnesses were caused by circulatory problems. Spinning and swinging his patients for hours, he thought, helped to reduce blood flow to the brain and lower the pulse. Bloodletting, another of Dr. Rush's unusual treatments, was perceived to beget healthy circulation. Mentally ill were believed to be unable to feel hot or cold temperature and were kept chained in unheated hospital cellars, cages, and slept on the floor. These institutions were called asylums; patients there were hardly clad in any clothes, were fed unsanitary food and kept hungry. Women, considered to be inferior to men, were treated even worse. Females tried to hide their problems out of fear to be stigmatized as mentally ill and thus be treated poorly and harshly.

This approach changed only in the late 18th century, when the French physician Philippe Pinel introduced treatment programs in the hospitals in an attempt of improving conditions in mental institutions in France. The next step was made in 1883, when Emil Kraepelin, a German psychiatrist, suggested the diagnosis and classification of schizophrenia. He also for the first time suggested, that brain abnormality was the biological underpinning of schizophrenia, making the first giant step toward moving psychiatry under the umbrella of medicine along with other medical disciplines. In the dawn of the twentieth century, the famous Austrian psychiatrist Sigmund Freud proposed a theory of the unconscious mind greatly affecting an individual's personality and behavior, laying the foundation for psychoanalysis, taking Europe and other countries by storm.

As follows from this brief historical overview, mental illness has always been perceived as something dark, scary and mysterious, more as a curse, sometimes a punishment; but not an illness or suffering deserving help. Unlike mental illness which has been associated with supernatural forces and evil spirits, or presented as philosophical or spiritual conflict, other medical problems were explained biologically and treated with available remedies. Heart and lung disease had been known in 3000 BC and treated with herbs and garlic.

One of the explanations for such a discrepancy is the lack of tangible evidence substantiating mental illness. Signs of heart disease were found in mummies in 3000 BC as well as in the remnants of famous Nefertiti. We are short in the evidence department, when it comes to psychiatry. Medicine started as a phenomenological, descriptive field, which gradually turned into science, based on the centuries of comparing symptoms with outcomes, anatomical changes, and postmortem studies. Until the science gave us means to look into the human body through very sophisticated devices and see what was wrong inside it, generations of physicians made their diagnosis and recommended the treatment by talking to and examining the patient. Surprisingly, their diagnostic accuracy was high.

The biological origin of the body medical problems can be visualized, or touched, or physically examined, or looked at with the help of sophisticated diagnostic tools readily available in many different places. Unlike body problems, the changes of the brain happen at the molecular level, which cannot be detected right away, even with the most sophisticated hi-tech equipment. Only over the last decade, imaging studies of the brain became more available. These studies showed anatomical changes in the brain happening in the mostly long course of depression, schizophrenia, or other psychiatric diseases. As convincing and consistent as those findings are, they cannot be used as early diagnostic tools to substantiate our findings or make the final and indisputable diagnosis. One of the common questions most of the patients or their parents ask me is: how come that if I/my child suffer from a chemical imbalance of the brain, you cannot order a test and show it to me? The truth is, that no such tests have any diagnostic value. Unlike the rest of the medicine, where a test may show what is wrong with the body, most of the tests in psychiatry at the very best would just confirm what areas of the brain are afflicted, without any benefits for the choice of the treatment or prediction of the outcome. Needless to say, in the time of managed care medicine, nobody is eager to approve any expensive tests in general, leave alone something of a limited practical value. This is the critical point, where the concept of a diagnosis and treatment choices in psychiatry become different from the rest of medicine, causing the lack of trust in the discipline. "If there is nothing to see, how come that it is a disease? Where are the objective criteria of the condition?"- patients tend to repeat time and again. At least some of the patients suffering from schizophrenia talk about their unrealistic perceptions, delusions, paranoia, and auditorial hallucinosis, show erratic and visibly abnormal behavior. When somebody suffers from depression, even loving family members request this person "to pull him/her together", recommend changes of life style, better nutrition etc. Unfortunately, depression is a serious medical condition, potentially ensuing suicidal attempts and death and causing significant changes in the brain: atrophy of a very important memory part of the brain (hippocampus) and other anatomical changes. Again, unlike other medical fields, those changes are more apparent as a result of a long standing depression, but cannot be seen in the onset. That's why we still have to rely upon our own diagnostic determination, including a thorough interview of the patient and the family, collecting data pertaining to any changes of life and medical condition. Every interview of a patient is a rigorously created set of specific questions crisscrossing multiple areas of life and exploring diagnostic possibilities.

The use of the first psychotropic medication, Chlorpromazine, in 1952, showed remarkable results in treatment of agitation, leading to a gradual reduction in the number of hospitalized schizophrenia patients. In 1954 the U.S. Food and Drug Administration authorized the use of chlorpromazine, helping mentally ill patients live more normal lives. Within 10 years, this drug was administered to at least 50 million patients.

However, many communities lacked enough facilities to help mentally ill people live independently. In 1963, the Community Mental Health Centers Construction Act was approved. It offered funding for the development of community mental health centers throughout the United States. The National Alliance for the Mentally Ill was established in 1979. During the last two decades, many scientists began to study the living brain of schizophrenia patients with a variety of new techniques, including positron emission tomography (PET) and magnetic resonance imaging (MRI). Using these technologies, scientists have found that schizophrenia entails problems in the development and chemical activities of the brain.

As thorny as the advance of adult psychiatry has been, child psychiatry remained even more "developmentally delayed". In 15th century literature, there was some mentioning of child problems mostly in the form of seizures, nightmares and bed wetting. Child psychotherapy was mentioned for the first time in 16th century by Heironymus Mercurialis of Bologna in relation to stammering. He discussed the unconscious fear to be at the root of the trouble. For the first time child psychiatry as a special discipline was mentioned by Johannes Trüper in 1892. Between 1892 and 1910 in Germany and France several books about child psychiatry were published and the term "child psychiatry" was used for the first time. However, Swiss psychiatrist Moritz Tramer (1882-1963) was probably the first to define the parameters of child psychiatry. In 1933 he identified child psychiatry as a medical discipline, with the same diagnostic, treatment, and prognostic approach as other medical specialties. In the US, Dr. Leo Kanner was the first physician identified as a child psychiatrist after writing a textbook, Child Psychiatry (1935). Leo Kanner was a medical graduate of the University of Berlin, brought to John Hopkins in 1928. Eight years later, Kanner offered the first formal elective course in child psychiatry. The first National Institute of Health grant to study pediatric psychopharmacology was awarded in 1960 and went to one of Kanner's students. The use of medication in the treatment of children began in 1930, when Dr. Charles Bradley opened a neuropsychiatric unit and was the first to use amphetamines for brain-damaged and hyperactive children he observed after an outbreak of encephalitis.

According to some historians, child psychiatry in the US dates back to 1899. At that time the first juvenile court was established in Chicago. In 1909 a group of socially active women trying to understand and explain juvenile delinquency created the first Juvenile Psychopathic Institute. The staff included a neuropsychiatrist, a psychologist and a social worker. Despite the presence of a psychiatrist, the main interest revolved around the level of intelligence as well as social roots and other socioeconomic factors, possibly affecting the formation of young criminals' mentality. This model was recreated later in child guidance clinics.

Child psychiatry from the very beginning grew out from the social environment, rather than medicine, becoming a focus of child workers in different areas, including education, criminology, psychology, but not physicians. Another organization, the American Orthopsychiatric Association (AOA), was formed in 1924. It was multidisciplinary, and focused on prevention of child mental illness, but its members tended to view diagnoses as hurtful labels. In 1948 – 54 child guidance clinics were created. They were mostly owned by local educational authorities and administrators and led by educational psychologists, teachers, and social workers. These clinics were not affiliated with medical institutions, using limited classification of childhood disorders and almost no research or effective practices. In 1943 a new syndrome of infantile autism was described by Kanner. Early treatment was based on the psychoanalytic theory and technique as well as play therapy with concurrent guidance for mothers. The treatment was almost exclusively conducted by psychiatric social workers.

On July 3, 1946 President Harry Truman signed the National Mental Health Act, which brought to life the National Institute of Mental Health in 1949. A part of the program was aimed at the prevention of child mental illness with the main focus on the quality of mothering. A failure to raise a healthy child called for the intervention of trained professionals; and they were growing in number. Some of the adult psychiatrists and pediatricians were converted into child psychiatrists through federal training funding.

As this brief historical overview shows, child psychiatry (as well as the adult one) did not start as a medical subspecialty. Unlike other medical disciplines, there was no search for a connection between malfunctioning of the body or brain and the psychiatric illness. The answers to the psychiatric problems were sought in child up-bringing flaws, deficit of parenting skills, harmful social influence, educational problems, etc.

One of the main incentives to see a doctor and get treatment is a fear of losing the quality of our life or the very life itself. Somehow the psychiatric problems are not viewed as such and are not believed to be life threatening, as malignant tumors or terminal lung or kidney diseases. Unfortunately, this is not true. Suicide is the third leading cause of death in adolescents (homicide being the second). So, what is suicide if not the reflection of mental illness? There is no breakdown data in the homicide statistic in adolescents, but mental illness definitely is one of the major triggers of homicide. Everybody remembers Columbine and Virginia tech school massacres. All three adolescents had psychiatric history and were on medications. According to the media, they were treated for "depression", but it appears, that all of them were either under- or misdiagnosed and undertreated. The result of that were the mass murders. There is a long list of school shootings both in the US and Europe, but the common denominator is the presence of mental health issues in the past or/ and at the time of the shootings. One of the adolescents, who shot his parents dead, later admitted to the prison psychiatrist, that he has been hearing voices telling him to kill his parents, which he did.

At one point of my professional life, I was involved with the forensic system treating, on the outpatient basis, psychiatric patients, who in the past had committed homicides. All of them were pleasant and ordinary people at the time of our encounter. In a matter of fact way they told me about their crimes - all of them committed because those patients were living a psychotic episode, hiding it from their psychiatrists and not taking their medications, thinking that they were not ill. They heard voices telling them to kill others, friends, family members, their children and coworkers. In all of them, mental illness either was not diagnosed or treated correctly, or patients stopped taking their medications and found themselves totally controlled by their illness. Since they were treated, they realized what happened, but it was too late to bring back those killed by them. Mental illness can be as dangerous and lethal as malignancy, or severe heart attack, and strikes people regardless of their age – young or old.

The demand for child and adolescent psychiatrists continues to far outstrip the supply worldwide. There is also a severe misdistribution of child and adolescent psychiatrists, especially in rural areas, where access to them is significantly reduced. I have met at different professional functions my colleagues, covering singlehandedly areas of hundreds of square miles in the capacity of both child and adult psychiatrists. They were not sure how many thousands of patients they had under their care and just shrugged when asked how they managed this huge caseload. There are currently approximately 6,500 practicing child and adolescent psychiatrists in the United States. A report by the US Bureau of Health Professions (2000) projected a need in the year 2020 for 12,624 child and adolescent psychiatrists, but a supply of only 8,312 predicted. In the 1998 report, the Center for Mental Health Services estimated that 9-13% of 9 to 17-year-olds had serious emotional disturbances, and 5-9% had extreme functional impairments. However, in 1999, the Surgeon General reported that "there is a dearth of child psychiatrists." Only 20% of emotionally disturbed children and adolescents received any mental health treatment, a tiny percentage of which was performed by child and adolescent psychiatrists. Furthermore, the US Bureau of Health Professions projects, that the demand for child and adolescent psychiatry services will increase by 100% between 1995 and 2020. This shortage of professionals along with the deep sitting notion, that anybody can be a specialist in child psychiatry, is causing a lot of confusion and pain for parents and their children.

Once, a wife of my colleague called me in anguish and through sobbing told, that her 4 year old child was diagnosed today with autism by a … music teacher. The child was not interested in learning a boring song and preferred to pay attention to his new matchbox car rolling it back and forth. It was enough for the teacher to state, that the child does not make eye contact, does not pay attention and plays by himself in a repetitive manner, meeting all criteria for autism, as she knew them. On exam, the child turned out to be a cute angelic boy, who started playing with me right away. He looked at me and talked to me, and at last whispered his biggest secret into my ear: he had "an accident" last night and was very ashamed of it. My diagnosis was "presumptuous incompetence" in the teacher and probably lack of music pitch in this little boy. It is not unusual to hear from a parent, that the child was "diagnosed" with ADHD by a teacher at school. It always puzzles me – why people cannot stick to what they are trained to do professionally? If we have a plumber in the house, he does not offer his services to fix our fridge or mend our cloths. Nor would we ask him to. When it comes to mechanics we trust professionals in the particular areas. A child psychiatrist has to withstand a stiff competition with multiple opinions of friends of the parents, who know somebody who has a kid "just like yours" doing so well on vitamins and special diets, or teachers at school, for whom any child not marching to their orders has ADHD, etc. Some Hollywood celebrities like Tom Cruz proclaim their disdain for ADHD (other mental illnesses are not even considered), stating that scientology is the universal cure.

The psychiatric diagnosis, especially in children, is extremely complicated and based on a constellation of multiple data. Even a school psychologist cannot make a medical diagnosis based on the result of a psychological evaluation. A psychological evaluation shows specific areas of deficit in attention span, or cognition, or memory, or any other domains of intellectual functioning. It can indicate changes of mood or level of perception, but cannot be used as a diagnostic instrument for a complex psychiatric disease. As a part of my work for the Board of Special Education I had my share of disagreements with some school psychologist adamant about having an upper diagnostic hand. They firmly believed that the lack of attention span detected on the psychological exam entitles them to give the diagnosis of ADHD. The fact, that the child was hearing voices or had other psychotic symptoms, controlling the thought process, totally escaped them. The boundaries between psychology and psychiatry got blurred to the detriment of the parents, who got confused, and the children, who did not get much needed treatment.

The boundaries can be further distorted by pediatricians dealing with children for their whole careers: some of them automatically write a prescription for Ritalin and such as soon as they hear "hyperactive" or "inattentive." It does not occur to them, that inattention could be a sign of something totally different and much more dangerous than ADHD. Luckily, some pediatricians are extremely attuned to any nuances of the child psyche and know when to suspect a psychiatric problem and refer the child to a psychiatrist. I sincerely bow to them!

Critics of psychiatry often argue, that psychiatric diagnosis lacks "objectivity" and "medical models", particularly when compared with diagnosis in other medical specialties. However, when one examines interrater reliability — an important component of objectivity, the agreement among psychiatrists for several major psychiatric disorders is generally on a par with those in other medical specialties. Nonetheless, in psychiatry, as in the rest of medicine, there is an irreducible element of subjectivity. That is part of the "art" of medical and psychiatric practice (Ronald Pies 2007). On the other hand, child psychiatry was criticized (especially with the growth of genetic studies, showing the familial patterns of different psychiatric diseases, especially schizophrenia) for neglecting the role of environmental, familial, cultural and other influences, undermining the value and popularity of family and individual therapy. Those critics state, that by discounting the psychological meaning of the symptoms, patients and their families forgo the sense of personal responsibility and expect to be cured by somebody else and medications, becoming dependant and losing adaptive and survival skills. The truth – as always – is in the middle. Let us look at an orthopedic surgeon – physical therapist – patient triangle model. The skeleton/bone problem is "fixed" by an orthopedic surgeon, who refers the patient to a physical therapist for a longer term care, but without ongoing efforts of the patient in following recommendations of his surgeon and therapist he/she cannot expect a good outcome. If any of those links are missing, the model becomes lopsided and is not going to work. The same is true in psychiatry: we need the medical treatment component, and the therapy component, and the patients' effort component in order to expect a better outcome.

—————————— Intermission ——————————

Several families have shared experiences raising their children with mental health issues. It is only through their stories that we can begin to humanize the grief, the sorrow, and the roads, that had been taken to treat a child with mental illness. While each story is unique, the children, that are presented, share a widespread range of mental health issues. Each story contains a common thread, where the parent knew that something was wrong, but could not define this "something". Each parent in her/his own way, shares the pain through the initial shock of the diagnosis, anger, grief, denial, and then the moment of clarity and acceptance. These parents have shared their raw emotions to help you, Dear Reader, so that you know, that you are not alone. And while the diagnosis may not be pretty, and the long term outcome uncertain, these families offer coping skills that they have learned along the way. What you will find is the hope, that with proper psychiatric care a child with mental illness can lead a better life. We invite you to join our discussion.

Let me introduce our panel of mothers, taking over our discussion: Mrs. L. Anderson, Mrs. L. Hamilton, Mrs. C. Lawson, Mrs. L. Mariebelle, Mrs. B. Mertz, and Mrs. T. Strom.

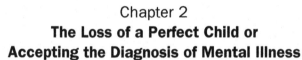

Chapter 2
**The Loss of a Perfect Child or
Accepting the Diagnosis of Mental Illness**

Mrs. **Merz**: When I was reading about this little boy and his parents, grieving the loss of the "Perfect Child," I thought about my own experience.

The loss of the "Perfect Child" can be a powerful and devastating experience, particularly if that loss reoccurs like a broken record, when you least expect it and can't control it from erupting into your life like a volcano. This is the story of my personal experience of chronic sorrow, my thoughts and insights to better understand the phenomenon known as chronic sorrow.

Chronic sorrow was introduced into the literature more than thirty years ago to characterize the recurring waves of grief, observed in parents of children with mental deficiencies as they struggled to cope with the loss of a "perfect child."

The words: the loss of a "perfect child," stuck in my throat as I read the first sentence in the article I was preparing for my class (I am a nurse). Overwhelming sadness filled me. My throat began to close up with a dry and horribly hollow empty sensation. So intense was the feeling, that I stopped reading. I couldn't even make it to class that night: halfway my stomach went into knots and tears just streamed down my face. I gave up. I turned the car around and went home. Even now, months later, having procrastinated by far too much, as I am trying to finish writing about it, I am still getting a visceral effect. Why am I so emotional, what is it in those words: loss of the "perfect child" triggering such an unforeseen response in me? At the time I didn't have any better words to describe this upsetting reaction, other than "depression." Now I understand: the emotional impact I felt was a phenomenon known as chronic sorrow.

You'd think my son is dead. He is not; he is with us and has survived to be nineteen. He is a tall, handsome and healthy young man who makes me proud. As a little boy he was sweet, blonde, blue eyed, with cupid bow lips, mischievous and daring, all rolled up in snails and puppy dog tails. To me, his mom he was an Arian Angel delight, perfect in every way, shape and form.

It was in kindergarten that things first seemed to go wrong. He couldn't write his name or draw. He had trouble reading. Otherwise he was articulate and bright, verbally aware and exceptionally astute. The teachers called it "Learning Disability." My little boy, who otherwise seemed perfectly normal, had to struggle to learn to read and write. We tried to do everything we could think of to help him to adapt to this invisible flaw. We arranged for tutors every summer and extra help during the school year. We tried every strategy suggested, always looking to find the right magic bullet to make it all better. We purchased all sorts of equipment, toys, computers, anything to help turn the difficulty of the learning process into fun. It wasn't fun. He got frustrated, angry, anxious and depressed. But he kept right on persevering, doing what the teachers suggested, trying time and again. For years I have had to watch him struggle and suffer with failures and with the loneliness of being different, then other kids his age.

Once I was furious with him for destroying all my Post-It notes and note pads in the house. Every time I wanted a clean sheet of paper I found a series of little drawings choreographed into a flip cartoon, moving across the edges of my pads. Then it dawned on me – he was teaching himself to draw in a three dimensional process! His brain wasn't wired to be linear. A pencil and a plain flat piece of paper created a huge stumbling block in his mind. He once told me: he felt his brain was operating in a snow storm, and his job was to shovel all the pathways for the neurons to go, where they needed to go. My heart bled each time I realized how valiantly he fought daily to accomplish what came so naturally and easily to others. It is the loss of normalcy that became painful, and with it - the ever present feelings of helplessness and hopelessness, because this struggle was never going away. It got even worse in high school, when the additional label of ADHD (Attention Deficit Hyperactivity Disorder) was added to his self identity. He hated the word "special," because being in special education classes only made him more different; when all he desperately wanted was to be simply the same. Our whole family dynamic was disrupted by this ongoing experience. Differences of opinions of how to cope with, or deal with my son's learning challenges caused added stresses and strains on our little family unit. Life's milestones of passing to the next grade and graduating from high school did us all in. The task of going to college turned out to be too much of a mountain to climb. When all of our friends were talking about visiting colleges for their sons and daughters, we were dealing with disappointments and making tough choices about whether adding daily medications is right and safe for my son's health and wellness.

These types of occasions filled me with a tremendous sense of injustice. The knowledge, that my son is very brilliant and very capable is diametrically opposed to his own sense of self, as being "stupid and different" (i.e. "not normal"). The more I tried to change his mindset, the more rebellious he would become. Feelings of rage, anger, frustration, fear, helplessness - all rolled in on me, like uncompromising pounding surf. Knowing, that there is no end in sight and no resolution other than to continue to persevere, became my chronic sorrow. And always there was the unknown question: to what end?

Since the 1960's the original concept of chronic sorrow evolved to include the following characteristics:
1) A perception of sadness or sorrow over time in a situation with no predictable end.
2) Sadness or sorrow, that is cyclic or recurrent.
3) Sadness or sorrow, that is triggered internally or externally and brings to mind a person's losses, disappointments, or fears.
4) Sadness or sorrow, that is progressive and can intensify.

Also different negative emotions like fear, helplessness, anger, frustration and other characteristic of grief have been validated by other researchers as being parts of the chronic sorrow experience.

Chronic sorrow differs from regular depression, because it has a never-ending nature to the experience of loss (or more correctly the ongoing disparity created by the loss experience), which prevents resolution of the grief. One of the researches indicated: "Disparity is created by lost experiences, when the individual's current reality differs markedly from the idealized; when the loss creates a gap between the desired relationship and the actual one." Chronic sorrow is also characterized by unexpected episodes of re-grief, which are triggered by simple events. Depression, as we know it, differs from chronic sorrow, because chronic sorrow is viewed as a normal response to losses. Chronic sorrow is not consider pathological or a chemical imbalance within the body. Still, the best way to help is to provide support in a similar fashion as to those, who suffer from depression, especially by fostering positive coping strategies.

Knowing, that my chronic sorrow is considered a normal response to a loss and not a pathological disease, was a comfort to me. It was also a challenge to the rehab nurse in me, to find a way to make the unexpected reoccurrences of chronic sorrow less debilitating and hopeless. Interestingly, one of the definitions of chronic illness as progressive, periodic and permanent - mirrors the experience of chronic sorrow. Knowing chronic illnesses within a rehabilitation philosophy, gives me an insight to the possibility of developing needed alternative models of loss, which could be based on the term "acceptance," or changing perspectives, or the normal physiological response to joy.

Why didn't we rejoice more in the triumph of my son's achievement of getting to graduation? Because we were too beat up by the war? Because the sense of sorrow and our perceptions of "loss of the perfect child?" We didn't allow ourselves to fully appreciate the fact, that he should have been given the purple heart of courage award for his monumental efforts to reach his graduation. He did walk across that stage just like everyone else in his blue cap and gown. That thought gave me great pleasure and joy as it should. And for the boy, becoming a man, it meant, that with his extra effort he could conquer college too, should that be his intention.

On that night on my way to class my severe emotional reaction, my chronic sorrow episode wasn't just about my son. It was in part a chronic sorrow that had morphed into something more, than the original event, or circumstances, that stole away the normalcy of my life and my son's life. Chronic sorrow became infectious and progressed insidiously and stealthy, like a diseased spore, hiding in my blood stream, waiting for the advantageous moment to break out and strike.

My tears were not only about my son, but also about myself. I have recently been diagnosed with a chronic disease and, because of my difficultly in staying on target and focusing on school work, I have been dealing with the realization I may be a part of the hereditary link to my son's learning challenges. So, part of the loss I was feeling that night was also the loss of my own internal "perfect child". It became a loss of me, as well as him, and filled me even more with that pervasive feeling of sadness. By nature I am inherently a survivor, and nurtured by my own parents to be a survivor (as many of us are) - to adapt to the challenges of stresses and adversities in order to conquer them. I can't put up with the idea of forever being a "victim," or accepting a victim mentality. The mental image I see in my mind's eye is that of being trapped in the never ending loop, like Sisyphus forever pushing the rock up the hill only to be beat back down again, and again: an endless victim of chronic sorrow. Being trapped and held hostage by your own perceptions of loss does not allow finding escape. And I don't like being robbed of joy. Joy of individual triumph and joy of celebration of success was a part of what we lost.

No one wants to be a victim, or lose the feelings of joy and normalcy of a happy and healthy life. Our options to develop a whole new way of understanding chronic sorrow perhaps need to be focused on a whole paradigm shift, away from what we generally associate sorrow with, the "grieving process" defined by Elizabeth Kubler-Ross, the creator of the Grief Cycle, with the five stages of grief: denial, anger, bargaining, depression, acceptance.

After all, we are not alone in our suffering, other parents and people, who have experienced a loss or losses, need to find healthy coping methods to persevere. All of us have varying degrees in severity of these losses and the intrinsic unending harm they cause in our lives. It is how we individually perceive the scope of that "chronic sorrow" and see acceptance of it. We can see it as a miserable end, a finality to give up on. Or we can cut our Shakespearian bow strings and see acceptance as a realization of a fact, with an intellectual view the pros and cons. In this case we can move forward with a plan of action and adapt in the best possible way to the "imperfections" we perceive and thus make life normal again.

"This is the very perfection of a man, to find out his own imperfections." (Saint Augustine)

Dr.A: How very true. Chronic sorrow is a devastating feeling, but can turn into a surviving mechanism. Beside the true loss of our dreams, hopes and aspirations, the initial "bomb shell shock" reaction is augmented with the system, which is not equipped to deal with children not fitting into the cookie cutter mold. Paradoxically I watched similar problems with gifted children, not fitting into the system because of their exceptional abilities, and getting traumatized by being thrown out of the conventional system. Children with emotional problems often get a label of being "incapable", or "stupid", or poorly behaved, getting punished for something they are not in control of. The next step after getting the diagnosis is finding a doctor and a therapist as well as the right placement for the child.

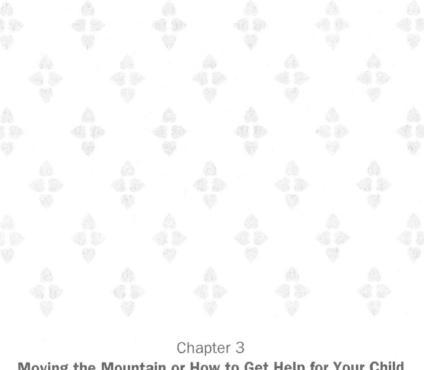

Chapter 3
Moving the Mountain or How to Get Help for Your Child

Mrs. Anderson: You have to find a voice to advocate for your child. There is an ongoing balancing act between the sorrow and the action! This is excruciatingly painful to come to realization, that first, a child has the illness nobody can see, or have a test for, and second, there is no help, unless parents become advocates (at times aggressive) for their children. Please read the following story as the Anderson Family navigates their way through each roadblock with family, friends, the education system, and medical community. The road is extremely tough, but as you read, you will find insight on how to raise your voice loudly to procure needed services for your child.

The Anderson Family story
As I sit here writing about our family, I am wretched with heartache and sorrow, as I watch my 13 year old son go through the agony of puberty. As his hormone levels have changed with this onset, his medications have stopped working. We are entering our fourth month of trial and error with medications to stabilize irrational and unsafe behaviors. We have put all knives and scissors under lock and key, as when he becomes severely agitated he threatens to kill himself. He has it all worked out. It is very scary, and we cannot take him outside of the house as we never know, when a volcanic eruption would occur. Our family is trapped inside as well, being held hostage to a raging manic control freak, ready to call 911. We do not want to call 911 as we know what will happen in the emergency room, and it will only send him into a deeper rage. We know that it will take time to determine a new "cocktail" of medications to stabilize his mood. And we know that he has no control of any of these behaviors. He knows that he is trapped as well, as his mind and body are not working in coordination. When he is having a good day, he is hyper focused on writing, creating board games, 3-D structures with computer programs, and talking obsessively about opening a restaurant when he grows up. But we sit in vigil, not being able to concentrate on any family, or household task, listening, waiting for the raging and frustration to begin.

Last night he stood in front of me, flailing his arms in rage and anger at a thought totally unrelated to the event that had caused this particular eruption. He was pacing, screaming, telling me how he wanted to kill his brother, how he wished he had never made a "game" deal with his brother that was made years ago, still crying and raging in front of me, words pouring out of his mouth making no sense whatsoever. In my mind, I back-tracked his every move and thought, that occurred throughout the day, to determine a starting point to bring him back to the here and now. The event, that brought this episode, was that the yogurt fell out of the fridge, as he was getting the milk, spilling on the floor. He went into panic mode, and his brother came to his aid, but told him, that he was tired of cleaning up his messes.

Back tracking, still back tracking, my mind concluded, that he was asked not to make a mess on the floor as it has already been washed twice that day, once from a syrup spill, and the second from a cherry soda spill, both as a result of his lack of coordination. In his calm state, we even joked about the clean-ups. Now he knew that he had spilled again. And in pure frustration with the yogurt spill, something that his body had no spatial control over, he had spiraled into an irrational shut down mode. He was angry with himself for causing the spill, and he was angry with his brother for harshly criticizing him. In his response to his brother, being mean about something that he could not control, he had called off the deal they made about sharing each other's games, along with the declaration, that his brother should die, of course, for making him feel bad about himself. None of these rational motives were clear to him at this time.

I pieced the separate stories together in factual order, teasing apart the two situations that were jumbled up into one distorted entangled mess. I watched his poor little mind sorting the puddle of confusion, slowly comprehending what I was telling him. I asked if he understood each part and watched his body movements calm down until he slumped into a chair sobbing. He looked up at me with his big beautiful brown eyes, filled with tears and recognition, and I gently reassured him that all was okay. I suggested that he was tired, and that maybe it was best that he went to bed. Good night Mom, I love you. I love you too.

Our two children are special needs children. Ben is currently 16 years old and is diagnosed with Executive Function Processing Disorder, Bipolar Disorder, Anxiety, Sensory Integration Dysfunction, and ADHD. Our 13 year old, David, is diagnosed with Autism/Pervasive Development Disorder (PDD), which includes a laundry list of autism spectrum disorders, some yet to be diagnosed, symptoms including components of Obsessive Compulsive Disorder (control freak), severe rigidity when it comes to food, resistance to good hygiene practices, not allowing people he does not know into our home, and ADHD. Both boys are also diagnosed with Asthma. David additionally has severe food allergies to peanut and tree nuts (EPI Pen on hand at all times), as well as severe seasonal allergies: the calendar can be marked as to the exact week each year, when he will be put on prednisone to alleviate the allergy symptoms. He is usually out of school for a three to five week period during the spring season.

On the bright side of life, both children are brilliant. And I say that not as a mother proud of her children, but as an onlooker, watching in amazement as to the verbal and analytical skills they both possess, displaying these skills far beyond their young years. Our job is to harness their major abilities, and to treat the symptoms that prevent them from progressing as far as they are able to become productive members of society.

The Early Years
Ben was brought home from the hospital on a warm summer evening. After the one allotted night stay in the hospital we brought him home and said, now what? I had been in and out of hard labor

for four days and was exhausted. None the less, we had this beautiful little baby to feed and love. Problems immediately began, where he wanted to be held constantly and would not sleep. He did not latch on for breast feeding, despite the several lactation consultants, who came into our home. We put him on formula, which he immediately adversely reacted to, and were forced to go to the "gold" formula (aptly named as it was outrageously expensive), which he spent the next 18 months drinking.

Ben did not sleep through the night until he was three years old. He would not sleep in his own bed. My husband and I took turns sleeping in the guest room. Ben was demanding. He would not take a bath or have his teeth brushed, and while we could never put a finger on any specific behavior that was "the" problem, we knew that "something" was wrong. We were challenged constantly by family members for our "lack" of parenting skills. When Ben was two, we set up a meeting with his pediatrician, who said there was nothing he could do, but he did council us to "never give up". He handed us a book on childhood behaviors, as we headed out the door. We left bewildered. Thus began our bookshelf of what was to be many more books to come.

When Ben was two, we decided to make baby number two. David arrived a month before Ben's third birthday. Where Ben had been our "nightmare baby", David was our "angel" baby. He smiled, he was placid, he slept 8 hours through the night as soon as he came home, and he had no interest in sleeping in the bed with us, preferring his crib. Ben and I bonded with David very closely, anticipating his every need before he needed it. We continued this non-verbal communication without even noticing what we were doing, until David turned 18 months. We noticed that he was not speaking at all. He also was not completing the baby milestones such as crawling or walking. And most important of all, he now became agitated quite often, crying and wanting to be held all of the time. Off to the pediatrician once again, where I was told, and made to feel like the silly dumb mom, that nothing was wrong. Just because Ben had started talking at a very young age (complete sentences at age 2), I was to not expect the same out of David. But there was no improvement and after several frustrating visits to the pediatrician, I was finally referred to a state program called Birth to Three. Many states have similar programs, stepping in to assist children with physical, occupational, and speech therapies in their early development age.

The therapists from Birth to Three came to our home for testing and immediately began a therapy program, which included physical, speech, and occupational therapies. David was far behind developmentally. A therapist arrived each and every day to increase movement and verbal skills. We kept a chart on the wall, listing each new word that David spoke. The list remained very small.

During David's first months of arrival Ben became excessively demanding. No matter what behavior tactic we used, nothing was working. I continued on with my collection of books of childhood behavior guides and would sit long into the night, searching information on the internet and landing at Amazon.com to order yet another new book. At age three, we brought Ben to a psychologist, whom I affectionately labeled the "kiddy shrink". Who brings their kid to a psychologist, and what can a psychologist do to work with a three year old? The visits were not for Ben, but for us, the parents. The psychologist observed Ben's behavior and would assist us in developing behavior plans at home. There I was, the diligent mom, every week visiting the psychologist with a stroller in hand, transporting David. Did many of these therapy behavior modifications work? No. But, they did indeed confirm, that I was not crazy, and that with continued diligence we might find the magic solution. Speaking of Magic, there is one book I highly recommend to all parents: "One, Two, Three, Magic."

I resigned my position as a Project Manager in the IT world when

I became pregnant with David. After spending my first pregnancy, all nine months, with morning sickness, I had no doubt the second pregnancy would be any different. In addition, I anticipated that on most days I would not be able to utilize day care services and did not want to add this expense. This was a wise decision, as I spent nine months in bed, unable to move from exhaustion and did not keep down any food. Ben and I spent the days watching ESPN and one movie, the only noises I could tolerate. I mention this, because after David was born, it became evident, that my husband needed to find a job with a much higher salary to compensate for two incomes. John was able to find such a position, but it meant 90 percent of the time on the road traveling.

When David turned two, I was asked back to my previous work position on a consultant basis. I found a day care center offering toddler facilities along with a full day kindergarten. It was then that we realized several issues with the boys. Ben, in kindergarten, was not writing or using his hands in any constructive form. Also, as in Montessori classes the year before, he showed no interest in playing with other children, content in being read to. David was having problems as well; he constantly tried to hide himself in cubbies and large play toys. I was called several times to retrieve him, as the staff could not seem to resolve his anxiety and crying. I once again resigned from my position so that I could stay home with the boys. With Ben's evident lack of fine motor development, I brought him to individual physical therapy. Once a week we would go to the facility, where he would work with a therapist with writing and hand exercises. Ben turned out to spend his time hiding under desks and equipment, unwilling to participate in the activities. Perseverance being the name of the game, Ben continued his private physical therapy sessions as he entered the first grade.

The Early Education Years
Problems with the school district started as soon Ben entered first grade in the public school setting. I requested physical therapy at

school as continuity with his outside PT. I was told that because Ben was participating in outside PT using our private insurance, there was no need to initiate PT in the school setting. Knowing Ben's sensitivities, I volunteered in the school library, David at my side, to keep an eye on what was going on in the first grade classroom.

As David turned three, his Speech and Language and Physical Therapies were now moved to the school district. This recommendation was not taken well. In a formal PPT (Planning and Placement Team) I was asked if I were to choose only one therapy, which it would be. The representative from Birth to Three looked directly at the school district representative and said they would immediately go to mediation unless he receives both therapies.

Ben was not progressing in school work during his first year. I continually asked for a PPT meeting to determine, if he required special services. I was told time and again, that this meeting would not take place. I began learning my child's rights and finally called the head of special services explaining my continuous requests and the principal's responses. A full five minutes passed after my complaint, when I received a call from the school secretary setting up a meeting time. During this meeting I requested testing for Ben, but was told, that it would be a bad move to complete the testing, as it would become a permanent part of his school record. I insisted, and upon completion of the testing another meeting was held. I walked into the room and was greeted by the school's special education representative, who informed me, that my son was an enigma. Ben was very bright on his verbal comprehension, yet, he scored in the lowest percentile on fine and gross motor skills. Special Education services began by the end of the school year.

As Ben entered second grade, David was continuing his PT and Speech and Language in the same school. I continued to volunteer in the school library with David at my side when not in class. I continually checked in on Ben's status in his classroom, where he remained at the bottom of the math chart the entire year. While he attended PT and OT, he made little progress in handwriting, gross and fine motor skills.

When Ben entered third grade, David entered kindergarten. I began to volunteer in his class once a week. David was already enrolled in Special Education and was given an aide in classroom. While I was in the classroom, David appeared to engage in class activities. However, in March of that year, I was informed by his teacher, that when I was not there, he was hiding under a desk the entire time. I was shocked that I was just finding out about this behavior! Another PPT was called, and we began additional PT and OT services.

Ben entered fourth grade and much of the same problems existed. We had finally started psychiatric services for Ben for his ADHD. In November of that year, Ben began to exhibit strange behaviors. He would walk the house the entire night and wake me to ask if he could have some food, bringing it to me, and asking me if I wanted some too. One morning I got up early and found the garage door open, and the loft stairs extended to the floor. I thought for sure we had an intruder and called 911. Three cruisers arrived with many policemen in tow. They all looked around and asked, if anyone in the house could have done this. As John was traveling, the answer was obvious, no. The mystery ended, when I questioned Ben that day, and he said that he had been up in the loft that night, checking things out.

During our next session with his psychiatrist, Ben was on the floor, rocking away, and spinning around, laughing at his antics. The psychiatrist called my husband and myself into the room alone and asked if any of our family members had Bipolar Disorder. I could count my mother's entire family, save for my mother, some having committed suicide, others who were jailed, and some just plain reclusive. John mentioned mental retardation in family members. The doctor informed us, that he firmly believed, that Ben was Bipolar, and that he was in a state of manic high. We were given a sedative medication and told to sedate him for a few weeks, hospitalization was not a choice. As we were in a clinic setting, we were offered very little support, only being instructed to appear back in a month for evaluation. We were in the dark knowing very little on how to treat our son. He was out of school many weeks that year and was diagnosed as a rapid manic case. Medications were administered, but offered little effect. We were finally told that he had to be placed on Lithium to control the manic episodes. We were never explained the side effects of medications, and it was a very frightening time for our family. The clinic however wrote a compelling letter to the school district recommending Ben to be placed in a different school setting, where he would receive the academic training that would assist him with his various needs. The district refused, saying that they had a fine program in place and do not need to provide a "Cadillac" education.

David was in first grade at this time and wound up with a teacher, who closed her door the entire day and would not let anyone in her room. When questioned about his progress, she said he was fine. Later in the year, an aide reported to me on the side, that David spent his days in the coat cubby area. I reported this to the principal and she shrugged the situation.

David entered second grade with full vengeance. He learned immediately that if he threw a chair at 9:00 am, he was out of class at 9:05. He left the classroom and tried to run home. He could not handle the noise of the classroom. I was asked to stay with him several times for the entire day, just so he would remain calm. He was suspended for his behaviors and made to stand in the principal's office for three hours at a time as he would not complete his work. His psychologist diagnosed him with Autism, yet the school would not accept her diagnosis. He was pulled out of the classroom, and ended up spending the rest of the year following the special education teacher around the school, as she checked on other students. I found out later this was in complete violation of his Individual Education Plan (IEP).

At the end of second grade, I fought for an aide for David for his third grade year. I was told he did not qualify for an aide, but the school would provide him with a temporary aide for his first three weeks to acclimate him in his new class. We disagreed with this plan and called the special education department, where we were told there was a special education program at the High School, a classroom for children with behavior issues from third through fifth grade. The principal argued that she knew of no such program, but the district told me it was available. I did not send David to school on his first day, and we set up an appointment with the program director and teachers to enroll David in this class. Annoyingly, it was only a half day program, but we were told that he would be ready in twelve to eighteen months to re-enter his regular education class. David stayed in the program for three years and allowed to continue until seventh grade. The program was not working, and it became evident that we needed to get him out of there. We also found out, that the program was set up for behaviorally challenged children, and that this setting was not in any way suitable for an autistic child. David's psychologist wrote numerous recommendations to modify the strict behavior plan, each time being rejected by the program leader.

We began to seek outside help for both children, as David was being warehoused, and Ben's needs were being ignored. By chance, and only by chance, we heard of an organization that provided Parent Advocates for children with special needs. Once our advocate began attending PPT's for both of the boys, the school district started changing their tune as they knew they had been violating both of Ben's and David's IEP's. Yet, no impacting changes were made to either of their programs. I ended up writing letters of complaint to the state board of education in hope of improving David's educational setting. Each time changes were made, but only enough to satisfy portions of my complaints. A very contentious relationship existed between us and the program, with David receiving the brunt of their anger by way of harsher classroom discipline. David emotionally regressed far back because of this treatment, and his psychiatrist wrote a letter to the school, stating that he was to be home bound tutored, until an appropriate program placement could be made.

By the time Ben hit eighth grade and David fifth, I had taken courses with the advocate group on how to advocate for my children. Lectures were given every week by special needs professionals, including lawyers and representatives by the State Department of Special Education. We were taught special education laws and the school districts responsibility to follow these federal laws. In addition, we were taught how to read and write an IEP, as well as different steps of taking on the school districts, when we disagreed with their program choices. It was an enlightening class to say the least, but I left it early several times in tears, disgusted and shocked as to how we had been coerced into placing our children in inappropriate settings, how we had been lied to about availableoutsideprograms,andhowourchildrenhadsufferedthrough important educational years - all at the ignorance of us as parents, and the manipulation of those same educators, supposedly dedicated to provide services to special needs children. I vowed at the beginning of that school year, that both children would be outplaced from the school district and into special education schools tailored to their needs by the end of the year.

It was tough, exhausting, emotionally wrenched work, as we knew we were up against the board of education, but we learned that knowledge equaled power and we forged onward, investigating every available program suitable for our children. I read case law on state educational hearings and the decisions on the hearings. I put all of the boy's documentations in order; so that we were prepared to provide evidence, should our cases go to court. John and I toured many schools across the state, reviewing program after program. The school district denied our requests for out-placement. Some of the special education schools allowed program tours only with letters of recommendations from the original school districts. We were appalled at some programs as they were just deeper levels of warehousing. We learned so much as we continued on with our mission! We ended up hiring an educational consultant to point the way for placement for Ben, and a lawyer, who represented us in mediation, where we were finally granted outplacement programs for both of our children.

While the road is still rocky for both, their special educational needs are now being addressed, and their diagnoses understood by truly dedicated staff. We know that as their individual needs change, adjustments to their educational settings will also change. It is an ongoing fight with the school district each year, but having come this far, we know that they will never bring the boys back into the district, especially after they have advanced so much in their new settings. I do have to laugh because at one point I disagreed with a situation involving one of the schools. I was pulled aside by an involved member of the situation, who told me that the school district warned them to be careful, as I knew the laws better than they. Two points for mom!

The Medical Community
If the school situation offered challenges, the medical community offered up bewilderment. Our first challenge was finding a new pediatrician. Both Ben and David suffered severe ear and sinus infections. We had our own room with our name on the door during the third shift at the local ER. Both boys' temperatures would rise to 104 and above. Aside from our behavior talk with the head pediatrician, I was constantly being pooh-poohed by the practice, when I believed something to be wrong. Through word of mouth we found a small wonderful practice in a near-by town,

where the pediatricians have been nothing more than respectful of our situation. My first words to this group were that I knew what I was talking about, and that they needed to work with me. We have been with this practice for ten years and all has been blissful.

When David was nine months, he began wheezing. The initial group of pediatricians, once again, sent me on my way, shaking their heads at the worrisome mom. I took David to an allergist, who performed a series of allergen tests. Immediately his arm indicated that he had an egg allergy, thus the cause of his wheezing. We brought the allergist on board and shook our heads at the pediatrician.

As the boys developed more ear and sinus problems, we enlisted the aid of an Ear, Nose, and Throat doctor. Ben had become a walking strep carrier. Adenoids and tonsils were removed in both of them. As part of David's increased speech and language issues, we also had to have several hearing tests. At the same time we had to have MRI's taken for his sinus problems. As we later learned, his sinus problems and infections resulted from allergies to mold, dust, dust mites, animal dander, and the many types of pollen in the air. We had to create a bubble environment to make him well. We laugh when we look back, as we thought this was a strain.

During these tests and procedures, it was important for all doctors to work together, each playing an integral role in diagnosing and treatments. Enter the psychiatric community: we did have the fortune of finding a very good psychologist when Ben was young. She left the practice group that fell within our insurance, to set up a private practice taking no insurance. This left us to find another psychologist. A large mental health clinic was nearby, and even though I was not happy with the facility set-up, we had very little choice. Ben was being treated for his ADHD by his pediatrician, so we initially went for psychological services only. As it became clear, that Ben was having additional troubles, we had an evaluation performed and enlisted the aid of a psychiatrist. Just as soon as we had begun to trust this doctor and believe in what he was saying, he left the practice for private practice, again, taking no insurance. We were set up with a new psychiatrist, with whom we had to develop a new relationship.

Ben's new psychiatrist began experimenting with many medications. We learned that a side effect of Lexapro caused uncontrollable bowel movements. Ben was in Depends for a week. I could not send him to school in Depends! There were many medications administered during this period making him dopey and lethargic. Again, I could not send him to school in these states. I was chastised heavily for keeping him home, and I argued back, that he would not be able to learn anything in these states. Sending him to school would only cause adverse attention. He was crying in school and ostracized by his classmates.

One day our clinic informed us, that they would no longer be treating private insurance clients, switching to state cases only, and that we had two months to find a new practice. Yet another frustrating search, yet another utter waste of valuable time. I began a search for a different group of professionals to work with the boys. We walked into countless offices, meeting up with the strangest of doctors. We left some offices wondering, what planet from they came, as we did not understand a word they said about the diagnosis and treatment. Some doctors were indignant. Other doctors talked down to us, others carried their ego on their shingle. We went to one psychiatrist who asked us to fill out twenty pages of information. This took hours and hours of my time. Upon arrival at the appointment, the doctor took a quick glance at the "novel" and wrote out three pre-dated scripts, one for each of the up-coming months for an ADHD medication, and told us to come back in three months. I was enraged, that he had the audacity to demand my time yet offering none of his. And we had to pay him. We never went back.

With a two month time limit, we ended up at the Children's Hospital Mental Health Department. Ben was assigned an APRN and David assigned a medical doctor. We arrived every month, often waiting over an hour for each appointment. We were very frustrated, as this was a terrible environment for kids with anxiety to wait for such long periods of time. At their appointments very little medication changes were introduced. The APRN hesitated each month to make a change, insisting that she had to discuss any changes with the doctors in the hospital. We had to wait another month to make any changes. For David, his doctor saw him for five minutes and then out the door, no answers, no changes, "it's all behavior." When we went to the medical community for help for their psychiatric needs, they were of no help to us.

In seventh grade Ben hit puberty. His medications were not working, he had several school issues, and his anxiety and mania soared through the roof. He went to school for several days and told his teachers that he wanted to jump off the school roof. The school treated this as a valid threat, and we sought medical advice from his APRN. She stared blankly, and finally made the decision to recommend admittance to the hospital. We had to enter Ben through ER, where he was evaluated for twenty three hours to determine, if he was in danger of hurting himself. Out of the school setting, he was not anxious. Therefore it was determined, that he was safe, and we were sent home. Back at school, Ben began his crying again, along with the jumping off the roof threats. Back to the ER, where he was evaluated again, and sent home again, this time because there were no beds available in any of the local pediatric psychiatric settings. Repeat performance, back in ER again (I took him earlier in the day), and, finally, a bed was available. It was midnight by the time he was admitted. We spent several hours admitting him, filling out countless questionnaires and medical history forms. He was inpatient for eight days, when the hospital called and asked me to come and fetch him, as he was too anxious in the hospital. His medications were never changed, and his discharge councilor had no offering of in which direction to seek help. She was condescending, vague, and useless. I left the hospital with Ben, raging at the system, having gained no help.

We were in search of a new psychiatrist. We came across two names. One doctor was a neuropsychologist, the other a psychiatrist. We visited the neuropsychologist first and went through two hours of questioning from inception to present. We became very apathetic with the family history routine by this point. She indicated that she could help us, but that she was not going to make any medication changes, and that we needed to come several times, so that she could get to know the children. This would take about three months. I knew immediately that I could not and would not work with this woman.

The next doctor that we went to was a psychiatrist recommended by our pediatrician, someone new that they had met. I was a little leery; after all, they were the ones who sent me to the doctor with the twenty page novel. We met with this woman, who quickly and accurately diagnosed the boys, went over their current medications and came up with a PLAN to withdraw them from their current medications, that were not working, and to introduce a series of medications that might do the trick. It took several months for Ben to withdraw from the Lithium, but as he was doing that, she introduced other medications, that calmed his symptoms right down. As with David, she accomplished the same routine. It took this doctor all of two months to put these boys in a place where I had never seen them. Functioning, alert, and, what's the word I am looking for – happy. A doctor had now come into our lives, marching us forward to finally be able to put them in a place where they could attain to learning.

I mentioned earlier, doctors need to collaborate with one another when working with multiple diagnoses. The boys were both on several asthma medications, some preventative, some fast acting like their rescue inhalers. During the spring allergy season, we would walk out of the allergist with at least five prescriptions for David's allergies. We soon found out, that the allergy medications interacted adversely with the psychiatric medications. The allergist refused to consult with the psychiatrist. After several requests with the allergist, we gave up and left his practice. We went back to the pediatricians' office and told them, that they were now taking over the role of the allergist. It took a lot of research on all of the doctors' part to find medications playing nicely with each other. We have found that some of the medications would interact for a few weeks out of the year and we just have to deal with it.

It took a very long time to meet up with doctors that we love and trust. This is not like taking a toaster to a repair shop. We are entrusting these doctors to care for our children: these are very serious relationships that are not to be taken lightly.

Home Life

I recently read a statistic, that seventy five percent of marriages with one or more special needs children end in divorce. I fully understand this statistic. My husband, John, and I are still married, because John travels full time, and we could never afford two households. We love each other, but raising two boys with complex diagnoses is a 24 x 7 job. The stress of raising our children causes a heavy strain on our relationship and offers very little time for a marriage to succeed. We know that we are in this for the long haul. Our constant worry is no matter how much work and effort we put into raising and finding appropriate programs and therapies for our children, we have no idea what they will be capable of as they enter their adult years. With each new diagnosis life became more isolating for our family. We thought David's peanut allergy, diagnosed at twelve months, was a truly horrifying thought. We learned all about how we had to change out our pantry and eating habits. That was nothing, compared to what was in store in the upcoming years.

We slowly realized that we could no longer bring the boys to church. I was volunteering as the Sunday school director, mainly, once again, to keep an eye on the boys. I also became the director of Vacation Bible School, thinking that this would provide an outlet for the boys to interact with other children. We discovered that the boys could not tolerate the loud organ music, or the chaos of the many people surrounding them in a large public area. I backed out of all church commitments, as they were not benefitting from these exposures.

Holiday traditions, as we knew them growing up, were a constant disaster. Again, as our families joined in celebration, both boys would be rocking away on the floor, ears covered from all of the noise and several people talking at one time. Family members would criticize us for not making them behave to their standards, offering good sound advice on how to straighten them out. I usually left these events sick to my stomach as to the lack of their understanding: they chose ignorance over empathy and respect for our situation. Over the years we have stopped attending such functions, including many important family events from the inability of attending with the boys.

We have also lost many friendships with neighborhood and relative's families. As their children grew in "normal" settings, our children fell back very quickly. It was evident, that we could not interact on a family level, and soon, one by one, we lost yet another relationship that would have thrived in another situation. It was a very sad realization on an adult level, as we, more than ever, needed adult communication and stimulation to keep a level of sanity. We now have very few close friends, mine being from women I have known for years, who accept our situation. John is without any close relationship, as his traveling prevents him from develo-ping any friendships. He meets new people in his travels, but there is no solid man time in his life. We can never have visitors over our home, never enjoy barbeques with family and friends, or have an intimate dinner with another couple. It is a very lonely existence we lead, especially with John being away so often. I do want to acknowledge my parents, who live right around the corner, as they have been staunch supporters from day one, and even though they had to come on board and be educated about the aspects of all of the disorders, they have never left us. My mom is my first call, when situations get out of control, her presence supporting me during the mad world our home can become, when the boys are out of control.

As I have said above, John and I share very little time playing husband and wife. There is always a crisis with school or medications that we have to attend to, never allowing for us to have alone time. Once in a while, my mom would stay the night so that we can get to a hotel, but we barely get to relax, and it is time to get home. Our escapes are always local. One morning, I woke up in the hotel room and could not fathom the thought of having to come home. I begged my husband to please call my mother to ask her to stay another night. I told him that if he called and pleaded, she would say yes to him. It worked and I lay in bed all day. Resting.

We do however; take family trips to local area hotels, and with John's travel points we are able to afford this luxury. We have learned to visit off season, enter restaurants at early low-crowd times, and to keep our activities low key, and in short time periods. We have also learned to respect the boys, when they say they have had enough, it is time to go. Frustrating as this is for us, we know, if we do not leave at this time, life turns to hell in a very short period of time. We praise them for their ability to communicate their need to us as it is the start of self advocacy.

Over the years we have come up with alternate activities to replace those ingrained in us from childhood. Christmas is very low key, very little decorating and certainly no sense of anticipation is allowed. We have developed new traditions, such as driving around neighborhoods, looking at the lights and decorations on the houses. John and I take turns spending Thanksgiving with our families, and we ignore all other holidays. Birthdays are kept simple, with a dinner out at a favorite restaurant and a special request cake. We ask them to choose one present, so there are no surprises and outbursts.

We even had the opportunity to go to Disney World. As David's medical treatment was addressed by a new psychiatrist, his behaviors improved. We could never have taken the trip previously. I cried with tears of joy, when at one of our first rides David was so excited and enthralled that he yelled "this is bloody awesome!" Every day at the different parks was an adventure that I never forget. The best thing about Disney is they have special passes for special needs individuals. This pass allowed us to enter rides ahead of crowds and avoid waiting in lines. We forgot the pass often and had to go to guest services to get another one. I arrived at the service desk, alone, as John and the boys waited outside. The gentleman was skeptical as he wanted to see the person, for whom the pass was intended. I pointed right out the window, and as if on cue, there was David, pacing in all his glory. I received the pass, smiling, as we were allowed one small bright advantage in a time when it was very much welcome.

Dr. A: Unfortunately this is a sadly typical story. You are certainly a winner as you were fighting for your kids and learning the laws, confronting the reluctant school staff to do the right thing. How many families lose the battle not having your knowledge, education, courage and perseverance! I do not want to paint all school districts the same gloomy way, but not many of them have appropriate awareness and means, not even mentioning the desire, to find the right niche for children with mental illness. I mean mental illness in general, regardless whether we talk about autism, or bipolar disorder, or schizophrenia, or learning disabilities, or attention issues. Usually any serious medical condition, especially psychiatric, does not start abruptly like flu. Even flu would have at least a day of what's called a prodrome, later crystallizing into a full blown infection. Psychiatric illness starts in an insidious way, with symptoms not intrinsically related at first glance or harbingering the coming storm. One of the psychiatrists (Dr. Harvey in 2007) coined the term "multidimensional impairment," quite accurately reflecting the complexity of the problems. Children from early age would manifest with different types of developmental delays – or what's perceived as such- becoming recipients of occupational therapy, speech and language therapy, psychological services, with no effect from either of those interventions. The Ockham's razor phenomenon comes to mind: where the term razor is used to highlight shaving away unnecessary assumptions to get to the simplest explanation. It means that *the simplest hypothesis tends to be the correct one and usually incorporates and encompasses different dimensions of the existing complex problem.* In other words, instead of treating children for multiple diagnoses (Ben has quite a few of them), it would be more medically appropriate to look at the whole "landscape" and think about the common denominator of multiple problems, addressing the root of them, not offering a dozen different interventions instead of one cardinal solution.

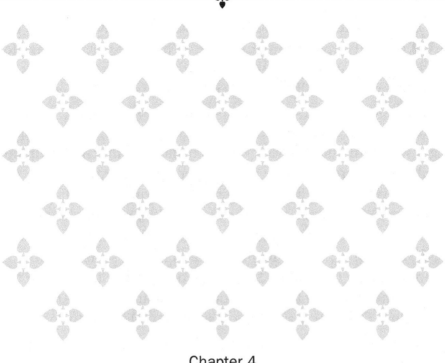

Chapter 4
Why the Diagnosis Is In the Eye of the Beholder or Medical Community – Opposing and Confusing Medical Diagnoses

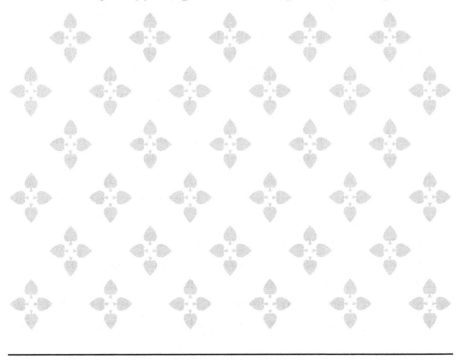

Mrs. Mariebelle: I do not understand why there is no consent between professionals? Why as parents we have to go through the ordeal of getting different opinions totally opposite and confusing? I vividly remember the evening in the psychiatrist's office. "Your son has a serious mental illness," she said. It didn't matter that my husband and I always felt something was not quite right with him; that we tried various behavioral therapies with no avail. These were words we never expected to hear. Or maybe we were denying it. I felt like my body had been ripped in half, and my feet were sinking into a hole. The upper half of my body wanted to throw up. "We could try a medicine called Risperidal," the doctor said. I couldn't believe it. "Risperidal? Isn't that for schizophrenics?" I thought, with my limited knowledge of psychiatric drugs. So we went home that night to think about it. And think I did. And think and think…Well, he was such a fussy baby…Difficult to soothe… requiring therapy for sensory integration…extremely limited social skills…

We started seeking counseling, when he was in preschool because of limited social skills. At one point, when he was five years old, we had him evaluated by a psychiatrist. "He does not need any medication. He is just a self-absorbed brat," said an allegedly prominent pediatric psychiatrist. Of course, we didn't take that doctor seriously, especially because his psychologist partner didn't agree with the "nothing wrong with him" part, and at least we felt we were doing the right thing with behavioral therapy. Then the psychologist thought he was doing fine and didn't need to see him anymore. So a couple of years went by. He was still challenged in social settings, had limited to no friendships, and a very low frustration tolerance. Then the anger set in. When he was about seven years old he became oppositional defiant to us. While he was fine at school and was no problem to his grandparents (if we weren't around), he was absolutely horrible at home. By the time he was eight years, he was so belligerent, especially with his dad, that we honestly thought he was possessed. No punishment worked.

No behavioral strategy worked. We asked the pediatrician for a reference for a therapist. The pediatrician questioned our need, stating, that he thought our son was just fine. We started therapy with a licensed clinical social worker with no improvement of behavior. So we asked for a referral to a psychiatrist, thinking maybe medications were the answer.......

Now we had an answer, but we didn't like it. After stewing about it and calling the therapist in tears, I decided our son should try the Risperidal. WOW. What a difference. I remember within two days on it our son said, "Wow! I can really concentrate!" He was much more pleasant with us and with himself. It was like a dream. But, of course, this was not the end of the story. After about two weeks of taking Risperidal he became very sad, weeping uncontrollably. He had to stay home from school. "This is what I thought would happen"- stated the psychiatrist, "we've peeled off the outer layer and gotten to the core of depression." So we added another drug, Lexapro to aid the depressive symptoms, and the drug Lamictal to aid in balancing the mood. From here we began our five year trajectory of trial and error medication management and therapy to manage the moods. We also began our ever growing knowledge and awareness of psychiatric illness in children and adolescents.

Our son is doing great right now at fourteen. He is aware of his own illness and understands the importance of his medication at this time. With the help of his psychiatrist he has been slowly weaning off of most medications and feels good knowing, that he is only taking a minimal amount at this time.

As parents we need to remain hypervigilant about advocating for our child. Sometimes even he doesn't realize, what may trigger a bad day or event, so we have to "be his frontal lobe" as I heard someone say. Focus on the positive. Be able to joke about some of the idiosyncrasies that your child has. Remember, most importantly: Psychiatric illness is on a continuum. There is no perfect mental health picture. Treat the symptoms and understand your child's illness.

Dr.A: I wish I could give you a good answer to why there is so much discrepancy between different psychiatrists and their diagnoses. In all fairness I want to remind you about "uneven" diagnostic and treatment approach throughout the whole medical community and across all medical specialties. That's how second, and third, and more medical opinions and consultations come into play. Still child psychiatry is quite outstanding because of the polarity of its verdicts. Nobody in general medicine or surgery would give a diagnosis of a "self absorbed brat" not needing any medications. I do not know a single medical professional dismissing patient's complains and sending him out of his office without offering appropriate help. Apparently we are paying the price for ignoring the medical roots of psychiatric illnesses, especially in children. There are generations of psychiatrists educated in the spirit of "old school," considering the family dynamics and intrinsic conflicts as the basis of childhood emotional problems. One of the oldest and the most popular psychiatrists I used to know, a walking encyclopedia of child psychoanalysis and personality development, never gave any child a diagnosis rather than "narcissistic personality disorder." It wouldn't matter whether the child was psychotic or acutely depressed: the diagnosis inevitably revolved around the child's "narcissism" and apposite behavioral recommendations. Eventually some parents started avoiding him, refusing to seek his consults or second opinions. This psychiatrist rose many generations of child and adolescent fellows, instilling in them the same repugnance for psychiatric medicine and aversion to medications. The situation is slowly changing to the better: medical mentality gradually penetrates into the field, shaping the minds, making psychiatrists search answers in biology and pharmacology. It is a slow process, but it has started. Meanwhile, mental illness, especially in children, remains not well understood. If professionals dismiss parents' concerns, do not empathize with them, and suggest "behavioral interventions" – what could be expected from general public perception?

Chapter 5
**Whipping Boys or Public Perception
of Children With Mental Illness**

Mrs. Lawson: Do not underestimate mental Illness and public perception: this is another facet of what our children and us, as parents, have to deal with on a daily basis.

"Mental illness is not something my kid can control. It's like having a broken arm. You can try all you want, but you can't will it back into shape."

I have used this sentence to explain my children's mental illnesses to many, many people over the years. I expect the question from the general public. Sometimes, they understand, sometimes they don't. And that's okay. Unless you're living my life with three of four children with various flavors of mood disorder, there's no way you can really understand.

What I resent, is having to explain to people, who should know better: medical and educational professors and family members. I should not have to explain that my son or daughter cannot always control his/her temper to the school psychologist or to teachers. But I have to do this, because much of the supposed conventional wisdom about how to handle kids with mental illness goes to behavior charts and telling kids to "learn" to make good choices.

Sorry. If my kids could "learn" not to be sick, they would not be on medication. If a strict routine of reward/punishment worked, well, then my youngest daughter who's attending a school for special education students would be cured by now, since she's been dealing with a behavior reward chart for four years.

After almost eight years of dealing with my children on a daily basis, I've finally developed a script. It goes something like this: My kids are SICK. They are not evil or trying to put one over on you, or trying to be difficult on purpose. Their brains do not function the way they should, due to some mix of chemicals and hormones that researchers haven't sorted out yet. Behavioral therapy helps them to recognize, when their illness starts to overcome their reasons, much as diabetics learn to recognize the signs of low blood sugar. But recognizing those signs doesn't mean my kids can control having the illness overcome them any more, than recognizing the signs of hypoglycemia help a diabetic's body produce the right amount of blood sugar.

It takes time to get people to listen. But I stick to the script and that's worked for me. The worst part is well-meaning family members. They love you, they want to help, but they don't understand. They might suggest a different way of dealing with the problem, or that you're over-reacting by providing medication, or that they'd do things differently by taking the child around to many doctors because surely, one of them will have a cure. They don't understand this isn't like one specific health problem that needs to be attacked and overcome with aggressive treatment. They don't understand exactly, what I deal with on a daily basis. What they do understand is that they're a little scared of my kids, because of their tempers, and they tend to stay away because of that.

This result in isolation, which is the worst thing those who love can do to us. We need as much family contact as we can get. If friends or family want to help you deal with this problem, tell them the best they can do is be physically present. Sane adults around are very helpful. Even semi-sane adults will do. That way, their understanding develops. You don't just tell them about the problems.

They know.

Tell your family and friends you love them and you appreciate them wanting to help. But unless they can spend time daily with the kids and by doing that form their own judgments about what needs to be done; they'll have to trust your judgment. It took me a long time to develop that kind of backbone. I don't know if it's helped the family, but it's lowered my stress levels.

There is no miracle cure here. No one knows what really causes this, though there is a heavy genetic factor. I am convinced their problems were triggered in some form by growth hormones. I certainly know that the menstrual cycle and its release of hormones affects their conditions.

Still, whether this theory of mine is right or wrong, the situation remains the same. The symptoms must be treated on a daily basis. There is only constant work, a combination of drugs and counseling, and taking things one day at a time. With children and adolescents, there is always hope, that they will outgrow it and my psychiatrist does have success stories. But "cure" is not a word I think about, especially after the first few years of hoping that the next drug that's tried will be THE ONE. It's like a bunch of first dates. You're hopeful beforehand, things seem to be going well, but by the time you get to the dessert, it's all downhill.

It is all trial and error, leaving me to constantly question, whether I'm doing the right thing, with worries about medication, about schooling choices, about discipline choices at home, and the future. I try very hard not to think of the long-term and concentrate only on the short term, otherwise I would despair completely.

I have seen huge improvements, especially in my oldest child. But there are no choirs singing or anyone screaming "Hallelujah!" at some turning point. There's only the day you turn around and realize, "hey, things are better."

Family Dynamics And How To Keep Things "Normal:"
Mental illness affects everyone in the household: the kids who are sick, the ones who aren't, and both parents. In my case, I have four children. Three of them suffer from one flavor or another of mental illness.

The first really hard hit to the parents is the initial diagnosis. My eldest daughter is now going into her senior year of high school. She's a great kid: bright, ambitious, open and good-hearted. I think (though she'd smack for me saying it) she's even starting to mature. She was anything but easy growing up. When she was a toddler, she never slept well at night or during naptime and she would wake with night terrors. She often slept in our bed with us until she was four years old. A few times when she was four years old, she got so angry that she literally trashed her entire room. She threw her clothes all over the places, made a mess of her toys and basically created chaos when in the wrong mood. However, these incidents were few and far between, and while they concerned me, most of the time she was a great kid, setting up her dolls to have tea parties, playing outside, making up stories, and doting on her little baby brother.

It wasn't until she was in second grade, that I wondered if something was seriously wrong. Her fits became more frequent, which seemed strange, because she was far out of the toddler stage. She was often overly emotional. I chalked it up to factors outside the house. We'd just moved, she started in a new school system, and there were the baby twins in the house, which added another stress. Then she started having trouble sleeping again. She would get up at two in the morning and make beds for herself in the bathroom. She had thoughts about the other kids being out to get her. Her moods fluctuated badly between being extremely happy to being extremely sad. And she started losing the few friends she had at school due to her quick flashes of emotion.

But it was the not sleeping for a week that finally convinced me, that she needed professional psychiatric care. That and a very wonderful teacher, who did recognize that something was wrong, and cared very much about helping my daughter get it right. The day I finally admitted I had a special needs child was hard. I was dazed for a while, overwhelmed, wondering how I could fix this, whether it could be fixed, and just feeling helpless. You want to make your kid better more than anything else in the world and when you can't, it's the worst feeling.

She's been under psychiatric care since fourth grade. The medication has not been a cure-all. The counseling has not been a cure-all. She continued to have good days and bad days, and her illness really impacted her abilities at school, both socially and academically. And, yet, the school refused to qualify her as special education. They gave her what's known as a 504 plan, which means they'll make accommodations. But that doesn't always translate to teachers who don't understand, because for every one that did, I've found others who would give my kid a hard time.

Still, it's a success story. She's an extremely bright student and she's going to graduate from high school with honors within a year. But there are times, when it's been hell for her and, as a parent, I could do little beyond sit back and watch her struggle with something she never should have had to struggle with. She's fearless, and stubborn, and I'm sure I would have folded if I had to bear her burdens.

What I know is treating this illness is two steps forward, one step back. As a child grows, her body's weight changes, and reactions to medications change. She gets used to one med, and it no longer has any effect. So you go on the merry-go-round and play catch-up.

I know my eldest didn't like going to school. I should have pushed the school officials to make better accommodations for her, to keep a better eye on her. Later, I learned that it's far easier to get the attention of officials, when your child is violent, as opposed to when your child is crying or sad. Because of the safety issue, they take violence more seriously. They should not. The sick child is suffering just as much.

We had adjusted to her condition, however, and things settled into a new normal for a few years. Then we started having problems with my youngest daughter. I recognized the signs faster, though, again, they didn't seriously manifest until second grade. A quick temper, a worry that other kids were out to get her and then, far more serious symptoms of waking up screaming in the night, trashing rooms, trying to throw things, yelling, screaming, toddler-style fits in an eight-year-old. There were days that I spent half the time holding her on the couch to calm her down enough to even watch television.

She didn't sleep through the night for six months. I didn't sleep through the night for six months. It disrupted the entire household, far more than my older daughter's problems had. My youngest heard voices, saw things that weren't there, and seemed to be disappearing into a world all her own.

Tossing around objects in class will get far more attention from school officials than crying at one's desk, or hiding in the bathroom crying. They're both symptoms of a serious problem, but the school is far more equipped to handle safety issues.

It was heartbreaking and painful for her and everyone else. I'm not sure how we got through it, except that we took things one day at a time. She was far sicker than my older daughter. It took us another year to get adjusted to another new normal: a special school for her, teaching the other kids to leave her alone when she was throwing a fit, learning tricks and distractions to calm her down.

I had some hopes that her twin brother, as her older brother had, would escape this genetic illness, but it soon became clear that he had not. Once again, just as things calmed down for the new normal, my youngest son began having problems at school.

On one hand, I was relieved that the symptoms were so mild compared to his twin sister. Mainly, his mood disorder is often pure mania: impulsiveness and anger brought on by a complete inability to separate word from action. He's mad and wants to hit someone, he does. He's embarrassed, and upset, and wants to run out of the classroom to be alone, he does. He thinks of saying something mean, he says it.

He's also extremely bright, taught himself to read at age three, and self-taught himself computer programming, and read at an adult level since he was eight. I think it's highly likely that his school issues aren't helped by the fact, that his brain is eager for something more challenging than his current courses, something that will trigger his brilliant mind. He's not good with structure, but he is good at investigating and learning things all on his own, in his own time. He can tell you the history of all computer operating systems. He can tell you about the history of various anime programs throughout the years. He has an incredible memory for facts, figures, and places.

I sometimes joke that he'll either be Steve Jobs or Ted Kaczynski. On bad days, I'm not kidding. Having three kids in the house with impulse issues often triggers fights that become extremely hard to calm down. The results are not pretty and make me into a referee doing damage control, rather than a mother. It became difficult to sit down for more than five minutes to eat. I had to stay on constant alert, lest one of them hurt the other. And I couldn't let the kids stay at home alone together, as the older two grew old enough to babysit.

And while the three kids who are sick had to struggle with their own issues, it also affected their brother. My older son, born between the oldest daughter and the twins, asked me one day: "Mom, am I the only one in the house not on meds?" I felt sad to answer him that, yes, this was true. I know it causes problems for him. He's embarrassed to have his friends over at our house, because his younger sister's fits are unpredictable. Because he is a very responsible kid, he learned ways that he could comfort his siblings, particularly my youngest daughter, and calm her down. He learned to fly under the radar and not cause trouble because he was afraid I had too much to do already, and he didn't want to add to the burden. He had to endure watching his younger sister throws fits in stores and saw everyone staring. He had to endure being pestered by his older sister when in a manic mood. In some ways, I think he worked hard to make himself invisible. The calm one. The good kid. The easy kid.

I had to work hard to make sure that he wasn't neglected. Just because he isn't sick isn't any reason for me not to take his requests and his problems just as seriously. So I've had to learn to watch him carefully and anticipate his needs, because he won't express them out loud. When he makes mumbled requests, I make him repeat them, so what he wants doesn't get lost in the shuffle. I learned to reward him for his good behavior. When I set up behavior charts one summer to ensure good behavior from the twins and the oldest daughter, I included him as well, and he earned the most money. Being a good kid finally was rewarding and, more, it was recognized as well.

I like to think it's helped him in some ways to be a more patient person, to be more tolerant of those who are different. He's also learned to have confidence because he has learned to cope with a rough situation. He's a teenage boy who really has no fear of talking to girls because, hey, they're just people. But I wish I could offer him more peace and quiet to go along with that. I suspect his mellow personality is ingrained, and there's not much I did to create it. All I can do sometimes is tell him what he's doing right.

And yet, there are things he would enjoy, that we don't do as a family because the twins or my youngest daughter can't tolerate it. Still, he doesn't complain or try to get away from us much. He's glad to spend time with his mom. He appreciates things. But this illness has affected his life a great deal. It may one day affect his life as an adult as well, especially if any of his siblings have mental difficulties as adults. He may end up being their caretaker in the end. He worries about having his own kids, who might develop genetic problems. It's not an easy thing to tell your son that, yes; he might one day consider adoption as an option to avoid having kids with this problem.

Effects on the Marriage:
Becoming a parent can be hard on a marriage, especially as priorities are re-arranged. There's so much to do that you find your partner getting lost in the shuffle.

With mentally ill children, this problem is magnified tenfold. They take so much time and attention, that the adults who are not sick in the house get pushed to the back. Part of that is inevitable, but it also leads to serious issues. We all need comfort and support and if we don't have any left for our spouse, it creates serious cracks in the marriage.

They say that money is one of the greatest stresses in a marriage, along with kids. So, that caused us a nice double-whammy. We had sick children that required expensive doctors and medications that are not covered by medical insurance. But there is no choice, children have to be treated. So, each month a new bill or problem would come up, and we'd go a little deeper into credit card debt.

At some point, it simply becomes so overwhelming, that the stress eats at you on a constant basis. And there's no money to go out to dinner, or even for coffee, or some days, gas for a trip to the park. You end up with two-stressed out parents in a house full of stressful things, unable to escape for any length of time.

It's a wonder our marriage has survived. Part of it is that we are both intensely dedicated to doing the right thing by our children.

Splitting up would just create a worse monetary situation. But beyond the practical, we do enjoy each other's company. We always have. So we try as hard as we can to find little moments, but with all the time and money constraints, it can be difficult. The only advice I have - try to find out what little things might calm your partner down and act on them without asking. Kindness and consideration can go a very long way into keeping a marriage together through the rocky parts.

Dr.A: From public point of view children with mental illness just misbehave. And parents are to blame for poor upbringing and lack of boundaries. Even the family members come up with good advice, not showing a lot of tolerance, or compassion, or understanding of the concept of child mental illness. The teachers, the relatives, the rest of the public need to learn how to trust the parents when they say their children suffer from mental illness, not from parental neglect or poor upbringing. Do we have any proof to present to "nonbelievers" in evidence of mental illness? Something like an X-Ray, or a blood test? No, we do not. Hopefully, in the future we will have it. But for now one of the main objective indications of the medical origin of mental illness would be familial pattern of inheritance.

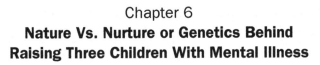

Chapter 6
**Nature Vs. Nurture or Genetics Behind
Raising Three Children With Mental Illness**

Mrs. Strom: Our three children ages three, eight and nine are under psychiatric care. Those are hard words to say and even harder to understand, if you haven't lived it. When we were approached to write our uncensored, honest story of ourselves, we wondered, what those words really mean to us and to those, who will read our story. If this had not been our own life, we fathom our response would not be unlike many people's. We guess that we would perhaps have shaken our head in judgment, disbelief or pity.

To fully understand our story, you would need to rewind ten years back. You would find a newly married happy couple, where life was good and on track. We were heading in the right direction full of hopes, dreams, and our joint agendas. Both college graduates, I was working as a R.N. and my husband, a graduate of Art School had recently landed a good job with our City. The pay was decent and thankfully, so were the health benefits. Outwardly my husband, Jack, is a big, scary, bald guy with lots of tattoos. His family knows him as a father and husband, who is sensitive, intelligent and kind. He is fun, outgoing, laid back, the eternal optimist and a fierce protector of principles and the underdog. We seem by appearances to be opposites. I tend to be introverted, type "A" personality, and am the proverbial "worry wart". Together somehow there is beautiful balance. Our family histories are uneventful. Hard working middle class Christian families absent of abuse, drugs, divorce or drama yielded good solid foundations; foundations we were eager to lay in a family of our own.

So, this brings us to the true beginning of our story. Years of irregular menstrual cycles and pain led me to the day I was scheduled for exploratory surgery for probable endometriosis. I sat on the living room floor and wept in prayer. Being a nurse and knowing possible outcomes of the disease, I grieved over a child I feared would never be. I turned over my anxieties and fears to the Lord and felt peace. Two surprising weeks later surgery was cancelled as whispers of infertility and pain turned to shouts of praise for miracles, cribs and nurseries. Against all odds, without surgery, I was pregnant.

Matthew's personality was strong even in pregnancy, like a shadow of things to come. Extreme nausea that never relented gave way to circulation issues and dangerously elevated blood pressure. I had to leave work as preeclampsia led to an emergency induction at 38 weeks. A short delivery of only three hours surprised the doctors, and medication meant not to be administered close to delivery sent Matthew to the NICU with respiratory distress after birth. He quickly recovered though and off we went into parenthood!

In reminiscing over that time, we recall our earliest fears that our children would inherit Jack's learning disability. Dyslexia had led his mother to become a strong advocate with the school system. She died when he was seventeen of a heart attack, but left a legacy of love and advocacy for her child. I feared I could never be like her – fighting school boards, laws and advocating. Little did I know at that time that I wouldn't have to be like her, I would perhaps have to be far more….

A word, that describes that first year, was "hard". "It's not supposed to be this hard," we would hear time and again from my mother. My mother is a woman of deep faith, my best friend and a child care provider for years. She had seen lots of kids of all temperaments, backgrounds and ethnicities. Her words echoed throughout that first year. Matthew had an undeveloped stomach valve, and our world became a blur of severe colic, vomit, specialty formulas, tests and specialists. Warnings came from the OBGYN that we may not be so lucky getting pregnant again due to my history. To our astonishment, when Matthew turned six months, we were pregnant again with our second son. Exhausted, but realizing it to be a gift, we praised God. Matthew was full of energy and walked early at nine months. By the end of his first year he had not had a single night, where he slept through and didn't wake up. His first year had a fitting end as he was hospitalized with a rotavirus infection. Entering that second year, Matthew never took a nap past his first birthday and continued to rarely if ever sleep through the night. He was endless in his energy. Bedtime took two hours every night and he awoke long before the sun rose.

My second pregnancy progressed easier and Luke arrived, when Matthew was fourteen months old. Life with a newborn and a toddler with unquenchable energy was arduous. To complicate matters, we decided my returning to work was impossible. Jack was working eighteen-hour days full time for the City and trying to get our new business off the ground to enable me to stay home. Times were tense, but we dug our heels in and persevered. Two years after the story started, our business was doing well, we were renovating our home, and I was a stay at home mom. Pictures at the zoo and parks show a happy normal family enjoying each other and life. Pictures often only show the surface, and under it the storm was brewing. Odd seizure like facial freezing, when Matthew would get excited, led us to a neurologist. Back to the Children's Hospital for more tests, where Matthew was diagnosed with a facial tic. "Can something like that even exist in a toddler?" we wondered. It seemed strange and bizarre to us, and there was no treatment. We were told only to wait, and perhaps he would outgrow it.

There seemed to be no breath between problems. Matthew was different, unique, and amazing to say the least. As he grew, we saw mood changes that were sudden and extreme. He had intense bursts of anger. He saw people that no one else could and he began describing odd scenarios like the Kingdom of God falling from the sky, opening up and creating a new earth. He would tell us about how he would speak to an old man in white and "Jesus" who came to him in long robes. We were amazed and disconcerted at the same time. Uneasy feelings began that would surface time and time again over the course of the years to come. Tentative reaching out to other mothers, describing our experiences and concerns, led to quizzical looks and subtle withdrawals. At age two my mother took Matthew to craft classes at her work, and his art ability astounded the teachers. "He is beautiful, sweet and funny, but he throws tantrums" the teachers would report. It went beyond tantrums though. He would fly into unpredictable, explosive rages, where he would kick, and wail, and throw himself on the ground for reasons only known to him. During these episodes he was impenetrable to even be comforted. "All kids have their moments" other mothers watching would encourage, but I wanted to yell that this was more than moments. Matthew was a whirlwind of emotions and after he exploded he seemed relieved and happy while we were left feeling spent and drained.

Jack and I breathed sighs of relief at Luke's "normalness". His energy was a little extreme, but we preferred to say he was "enthusiastic". When we found him standing on our kitchen table literally swinging from the light fixture, the pediatrician suggested keeping a small outdoor play-scale in the house, so he would have something appropriate to climb on. He walked at eight months, even earlier than Matthew, and although he didn't sleep every night through, his sleep was more normal. Overall, Luke seemed healthy, happy and easier going. He was inquisitive, and didn't seem to have the extreme mood fluctuations and anger that Matthew displayed. They played together constantly, but Luke often suffered from Matthew's quick temper. Constant supervision was necessary between them, especially as Matthew began to hit and bite when he became enraged.

Matthews Pre-K was a string of parent's nightmares. "Matthew threw a shoe at someone," Matthew bit someone," "Matthew ripped everything off the bulletin board." As other parents listed briefly at Parent Teacher Conference of their child's progress, we would hear echoes of our own fears. "He's brilliant, smart and fun. We love the excitement he brings to the class." But, it was tempered with "sometimes he gets so angry and rages. We can't predict it, redirect or control him." We too felt helpless to predict or stop his anger. We read books about spirited children and raising strong willed boys. TV was limited. We instituted constructive time out corners, good behavior reward charts and progressive loss of disciplines. We made sure the methods at home were followed at school. Discipline during his rages further incited him, and we followed steps to manage "difficult" children. Anger was something foreign to me. My husband, having a history of hot-headedness, related more to Matthew. "He's responding to being frustrated over something" he would relate. "He just needs to mature and grow out of it." We don't speak harshly to one another in our family, and Matthew's outward display of anger puzzled me. I usually received the brunt of Matthew's tantrums as Jack worked evenings. Jack though had to field the tearful panicked phone calls as I would routinely call him with reports of lamps being thrown at me, chairs being knocked over, screaming, biting, and fury. These rages though were mixed with one of the sweetest loving children you have ever met. He loved to help and was so proud when his behavior was good. When the waters were calm, he was caring and easy to love. During those moments, I could almost convince myself everything was going to be O.K. Love can conquer anything I thought. We began researching nutritional deficiencies, diet changes, and began homeopathic remedies for anger management in children. Our thoughts on medication were unified; natural product aside, we discussed that we would not be one of "those" parents who medicated their kids just to keep them quiet. I look back and see the self righteousness of our own words. A lesson of humility was beginning in our lives even at that time.

Luke's reports at Pre-K were like the ones we had envied for Matthew. Yes, they were laced with words like "super high ener-gy" and "ants in his pants," but what three- year- old could sit still, we wondered? Luke was sweet and extremely sensitive. He was cautious with strangers, but had no fear on playgrounds. He was always the child, who would find some unique, unconventional and perhaps not so safe use for a piece of playground equipment. He would always leap before he looked so to speak.

Our search for other families struggling with situations similar to ours continued at that time. Even though we weren't sure what was exactly happening, we recognized Matthew seemed unique and different from his peers. We continued to reach out to our church community, but withdrew as we saw the families with kids, who could sit quietly in the pews. I often turned inward in my prayers and reflections. Even when I would talk with other mothers, friends and family, I began to feel avoided. Other mothers had problems of their own and wanted simple play dates and coffee. It became obvious they did not want my ramblings about rages and fears compounding their own burdens. No one except my own mom seemed to relate. She was over all the time and saw our life with our boys. She would help with the dishes, laundry, whatever I couldn't get to due to dealing with tantrums or pure exhaustion. It was her way of helping when there was really nothing else that could be done. We would discuss Matthew's odd behaviors and anger, and Luke's impulsiveness and hyperactivity. There were no answers, but at least she became my sounding board. Mostly she would just listen, clean and pray.

Moving forward over the next year brought more of the same. During Pre-K Matthew's violent temper tantrums now became verbalizations. He opposed going to school one morning, and told me he was going to kill me and cut me until I bled. I cried quietly as I drove him to school. I often had to pick him up early, because he had acted out during class. We were doing everything we knew to do, but we were becoming aware that something was terribly wrong. Our pediatrician was at a loss, as we struggled to verbalize our frustrations and ever mounting concerns. "He'll probably grow out of it" he said, "Sometimes these things just work themselves out". He gave general tips on discipline. We didn't blame him for not having the answers to what was a difficult situation. We felt helpless on how to say "we need more help than that."

As Pre-K was ending and I braced myself every time I picked him up for the quiet "Can I speak with you privately?" I would ignore the other parents with downward glances as they quickly ushered their "normal" kids out so we could talk. That day did not disappoint. "I'm afraid he will be red flagged once he hits kindergarten" the teacher said in a hushed voice. He had threatened to bomb the school, when a project did not go his way. My heart sank and fear rose. I could feel her words coated with sympathy, but underneath I could only imagine what she was thinking. She didn't accuse or blame me, but I remember rambling, as my heart felt I needed to defend me and my family. My words sounded empty as I struggled to explain, that he was never verbally or physically abused. I tried to explain, that we didn't understand where he ever heard the things he said. He had no access to computers, video games, and only limited kids programming on TV. She nodded in understanding, but I remember thinking she was judging me, critiquing my words. I realized that perhaps it was not her judging me, but echoes of my own fears and judgments on myself. I wondered what we were doing wrong as parents.

We had no idea what our next step should be, but we decided, that knowledge is power, and we would not go to Kindergarten unarmed. If you have a plumbing problem, you call a plumber, but we wondered who in the world do you call in a situation like ours? So we sat down and thumbed through the yellow pages. We needed answers and we needed them fast. I called child behavioral clinics and family psychiatry centers. "We have a six months waiting period" and "Our minimum age is six" - was the common response. As the dead ends of full clinics and age restrictions grew, so did our anxiety. We finally found and settled on the first child psychologist, who had an opening to see a four years old child independent of a divorce situation. He was a behavior psychologist, and I was terrified of our first appointment. Jack was skeptical. I remember feeling very small on his big leather couch. "This is for people, who are getting divorced, do drugs or abuse their kids" I thought. At minimum I deliberated, that it was for parents who can't manage their kids. "We're good parents and a normal family" I recall thinking. The psychologist asked lots of questions and Jack and I answered as honestly as we could. Matthew's behavior spoke somewhat for itself. He climbed over chairs, knocked objects over, turned switches on and off and opened books. There was nothing sacred to him, and he had no boundaries. We continued meeting regularly with the psychologist. Meanwhile, I immersed myself in books on child rearing. I charted moods, and violent behaviors, and dutifully handed them over to the Doctor each session. I continued researching homeopathic "cures" for every childhood malady you could think of, but six months into therapy came the blow. I don't recall the exact conversation: "You are great parents; you're doing everything right, sometimes these things just happen, Matthew needs more help than I think I can give." He recommended we take Matthew to a child psychiatrist. It then hit us. There was no miracle elusive parenting mistake we had made. We could do everything to change externals but were powerless to correct something internal with Matthew. There is a stretch of highway along route I- 84 that has seemed to connect every Doctor we have been to. I see it in my mind, and that stretch of highway has come to represent many emotions to me. That highway saw the first of many quiet rides home.

The wait for many child psychiatrists who took insurance in the state was up to two years. We were appalled. What in the world were parents supposed to do while they were waiting? Everywhere I looked I saw "normal" kids as we tried to ignore bewildered looks from parents. One outing to the local aquarium produced those familiar looks from parents. They didn't understand why my son was screaming and pounding on the glass saying: "I'm going to kill all these fish; I have to get out of here!" We didn't understand either, and began trying to avoid any situation that might cause Matthew to become agitated and us - to be embarrassed.

Because of a favor called in by the psychologist, we got in quickly with a leading child psychiatrist in the state. I felt compassion for the parents who had no one to call for them. So off we went with thirty five minute car rides into the city and agonizing two hour waiting room stays to be seen each time. I felt badly for the Doctor. He would walk into a waiting room filled with expectant parents, tired kids and an armful of charts so high, he could barely see over them. His office was behind a locked glass door and then a locked wooden door. It seemed scary and prison- like to me. He was nice, and I remember he had pictures of his own kids in frames in the office. He looked as tired as the parents in the waiting room, and I wondered if he saw his own kids as much as he saw other people's ones. I wondered if his children were normal. We would prepare for days before those appointments. As parents we had to arm ourselves, because it felt like a battlefield, where we only had ten-fifteen minutes to cram month's worth of behaviors and concerns into a concise to the point conversation. Matthew was disruptive during the sessions: he would turn on lights, hide under chairs, and try to escape. (I began to understand the double locked doors). In the midst of all his behaviors though, Matthew's true self shone through too. The Matthew which delighted and amazed us, the Matthew I wished would always stay. He was angelic with fair skin, thick curly hair the color of corn silk and big crisp clear blue eyes. Matthew's personality, when calm and not enraged, was funny, sweet and personable. He was full of knowledge, and was charming as the doctor asked about school, and the "inventions" he would make. Matthew had increasingly begun "inventing". He would work furiously disassembling any items he could, and would go through our trash looking for new items to use. His drawings became elaborate, and he would fill long pages with hundreds of boxes and numbers. He never seemed able to relax, and would move from project to project from sun up to sun down. Wherever he went he left mountains of trash, papers and broken items. He would tell other people that he was a famous inventor and could build inventions that really worked. To watch him was exhausting as his energy was immeasurable.

As our sessions with the psychiatrist progressed, he seemed to like us. He told us we were good loving parents, and it wasn't our fault. We wanted to believe him, but we wondered what other explanation there could be? Loose diagnoses were mentioned, like ADHD, mood disorder, and possible pediatric bipolar. I wondered if he knew how parents hang on those words. They are diagnoses he might give every day, but can change a parent's whole world. Those were hard words that would come to define us, lead to anxiety, sleepless nights, and hours of online research. At this point we were exhausted, and worried, and we had to taste our own anti-med words that day, as we decided for our sanity and our family, to test the medication waters. We were blind sighted, as the first medication caused a severe reaction we had no warning of. The doctor's response was that he had anticipated the reaction, as it was a common response in mood disorder children. He said he had used it as sort of a "test". I could see my husband's anger and skepticism increasing. "Shouldn't we have been told that was a possibility? Our kid is just a guinea pig?" he protested. Yet when it came down to it, Matthew's ability to function at home and at school was continuing to deteriorate due to his raging. We both agreed what little options we had were running out.

I was pregnant with our third child at that time. It was a girl and a dream realized. We had discussed having no more kids, but left it in the Lord's hands. She would be our last child and I prayed "Lord, please let her be normal." It was a bittersweet time; a bright spot amongst turbulence. Matthew was five and Luke was four now. We began noticing that Luke made snorting noises and odd sounds that led us back to the pediatrician. "It's probably seasonal allergies," the doctor said. He had no explanation though for why Luke couldn't stand the feeling of clothes against his skin, and loathed anything but pajamas. The was no justification for why he wanted to bend his toes backward to touch the back of his foot, or why it would take 30 minutes to get his shoes to feel "right." He would cry that he had to flex certain muscles to have them feel normal. "Sensory issues are very common, and he'll probably outgrow it," the doctor supposed. The only thing the doctor could recommend was allergy meds, for the "allergies," which had no effect. Luke was very anxious and fretted over everything, which was so different from Matthew, who seemed to have no cares or worries.

As Matthew entered Kindergarten, we tried to focus on his tremendous strengths in building and drawing. Yet we found simple tasks like tying shoes and riding a bike eluded him. When Hope was born we were relieved that Matthew was remarkably patient and kind. He seemed to understand her fragileness and respected it. We requested a meeting with the Kindergarten teacher before school started, but she put it off. We tried to warn and explain his rages while keeping the positives in the forefront. "He'll be fine" she laughed and seemed confident: we were just nervous parents. Her laughing didn't last long though as Matthew began school and his extreme behaviors became evident. Academically, he was significantly behind in reading despite exhibiting great intelligence. The focus at school sadly was not his lack of academic progress, but behavior management. His reading scores were significantly below average, but the school continued reading strategies that seemed to be ineffective, despite our protests and concerns. We called meetings but the staff claimed they were bound by rules that discouraged formal educational testing before first grade. It seemed ridiculous to continue and waste time, as we saw him struggling to learn in a way that was obvious he found exasperating. Jack related to Matthews frustration. He himself was removed from regular education in third grade and placed in a special education school. It was at a time when little to nothing was known about learning disabilities. Jack's sources of school difficulties were severe dyslexia and dyscalculia, which were not discovered until Junior High School. His early years were spent in a program, where kids of all mental capacities and mental illness were mixed in with the learning disabled and behavior problem children. This environment created a volatile mix, where little was learned except survival of the fittest. He now harbored skepticism that the school system could do better for his son, than it did for him. We soon discovered there were overwhelming laws designed to protect the children. We also found, that this system has been created so complex, that nothing short of hiring an advocate or a lawyer can help the average parent to navigate them. Medically, Matthew was on a new medication by midyear, and we had a taste of two months of almost "normalness." He functioned well at school, and was pleasant and cooperative at home. It was too good to last though, and at the end of Kindergarten crisis hit. Nothing had changed, but Matthew spiraled out of control. Eruptions of physical and violent rages returned suddenly in school and out. He would run out of the school into the parking lot, hide under desks and threaten the teachers. By the end of Kindergarten, Matthew was being restrained almost daily due to severe aggression. The "people" he saw in visions, which spoke kindly to him before, became scary versions of people he knew. "I know they're not real because they are flat, and I can put my hand through them – they are really creepy and I hate them," he would say. We placed an emergency call to the psychiatrist and waited. Two agonizing days would pass before we received a return call. In that time came my neighbor onto the scene. She had two older boys, who had diagnosis, which seemed long and scary, but she was the first mother I met, who shook her head in understanding, as I spilled out my heartache and fear. She related because her family lived with the pain we shared. Her understanding ran deeper than vague nods of "I'm so sorry" and "I'll pray for you," and I believe that God orchestrated our meeting with precision.

Jack and I were scared and out of answers; she had the name of a good child psychiatrist. She was the first one to say out loud what we couldn't: "You are in crisis and need help." I didn't even know exactly what that meant, but I thanked the Lord for someone who at least was on the same road as us. The call from the doctor finally came in at 8 o'clock that night. The conversation was very brief, and he quickly suggested three different medications we had never discussed. (After searching online I found they were two antipsychotics and an ADHD medication.) He told me to think it over, choose one and call him in the morning with our choice, and he would call in the script. I was dumbfounded and Jack was furious. "Am I the Doctor?" he vented. "How in the world are we supposed to choose meds to give our son that we've never even heard of before?" he exclaimed. I stared in silence for a great while at the sheet of paper in front of me, all but blank except the names of three medications I had scrawled across it. I felt so emotionally drained that I couldn't even cry. In the morning we didn't call him, but instead called the Doctor our neighbor recommended.

So marks a new period in our story. Jack was supportive, but hated the idea of medications and still held out that Matthew would "grow up and out of it." He knew that the issues we were facing were deeper than behavior, but nothing he had seen so far from the medical community had convinced him they could do much better. Jack was reluctant to say the least to see any more doctors at that point. So, we began with a new psychiatrist cautiously and a little gun-shy but knew we needed some answers. I dreaded having to organize and present years of tantrums, rages, worries and anguish. The doctor didn't accept insurance in what seems to be a common trend among Psychiatrists. We could understand why as we saw from our own experiences. The previous Psychiatrist had accepted insurance, but we saw how the insurance company restricted and dictated sessions times and meds that could and couldn't be prescribed. Our insurance agreed to reimburse us partially for the visits, but we wondered how the average person with limited coverage could afford good psychiatric care.

So, off we went again with a 25 minute ride on that same stretch of I-84 looming ahead. In a marked contrast, we didn't have a wait this time. No crying babies or sullen children filled the waiting room. The doctor seemed fresh and eager to meet us. We shared our story and she listened intently, nodding in understanding. She appeared confident after reading our history and speaking to us that she could present a real explanation for what we were facing. She was direct, committed and confident. There was no vague hinting and we appreciated that. We left that day with a solid reality that Matthew had a mood disorder. The words hung in the air between Jack and I on the ride home, but there were no tears this time. There was only an odd welcome sense of relief. Perhaps we would finally get some answers. We may not like it we decided, but we weren't left to wonder. She recommended the book "The Bipolar Child" and we read it immediately. It was strangely comforting, like a video camera into our world. Suddenly we realized there were other people like us. We weren't alone anymore. Not being alone though didn't solve our problems. We researched and found we do have some relatives with one suspected and some confirmed mental illness cases. They are not direct relatives, but we figure our recessive DNA might just have merged to create a perfect storm combination for our children. We didn't focus on genetics long though. Playing the blame game on where it came from wasn't going to help us or our children. We continued with the same psychiatrist, and although resistant, Jack admitted that the medications seemed to be helping and the hallucinations and "people" Matthew saw stopped. I wish we could say that Matthew has been stable since, but we have learned that living with him will probably always be a challenge. Some days the waters are calm, some days there are slight swells and other times we batten the hatches for hurricane force gales. The last few years have been long and hard. Matthew is now nine and is entering fourth grade.

Jack still doesn't like labeling Matthew and is very skeptical of the medications. He comes to almost every doctor's appointment and remains hard to convince when a med change is made, or another medication introduced. He does admit though, that whether we like it or not, Matthew needs the medications to function. He is adamant that we try our best to only give the smallest amounts of a medication necessary for Matthew to function. Aside from meds, we have also learned to recognize signs, and watch his drawings and actions for indications of coming elevated mood. He still rages, and the bigger he gets, the more they scare me. He can be pleasant, cooperative and fun 98% of the day, but the 2% when he's angry leaves such destruction and turbulence in his wake, that it seems to overpower the good. We continue to endure the sometimes brutal medication changes and we know in our hearts there is no "magic pill", although I admit I still hold out hope and pray for it sometimes.

Our battle with the school system also still rages. We have become fierce advocates, nurtured and cultivated mainly by other parents and educators, who have treaded the long road before us. I find that it is hard for teachers and administrators, who are engrained to treat behaviors to understand anything different. I often lament, that it is not really easy to understand manual or guide to navigate the endless educational laws. The Internet can be good, but one has to be careful not to get lost in emotional forums populated by tired, angry struggling parents looking for the answers. The school held their ground that Matthew was in an appropriate reading program from kindergarten to second grade. They held firm that the majority of children flourish under the programs they followed, and to our amazement their testing of him showed absolutely no learning disability. It took a lawyer with a large retainer and a thorough evaluation by a neuropsychologist to prove them grossly erroneous. The neuropsychiatrist showed without a doubt that Matthew possesses a very high IQ with low academic scores, and exhibits significant academic learning disabilities. The neuropsychologist presented reasonable alternative ways he could learn, and be as successful as any other student, and the school was forced to implement them despite their reluctance. It angered us that the school was so resistant to change his curriculum and was not motivated by best interests of the child. It shouldn't be so hard for parents, and I wondered if we couldn't have afforded the lawyer, what would have happened? Despite all we have done to educate his teachers and those working with Matthew, we cannot count the number of times we have been called in to try to defend him and work out problems. It becomes very tiresome and burdensome, but we look now at the learning disabilities we had so feared when our road began, and they seem somewhat small now in comparison to what we generally face on a daily basis. Unfortunately the school system does not offer specific helps for children with behavioral manifestations due to their illness. So, he is currently in a special education program, mixed with mainstream for children geared strongly towards behavioral modifications. We fear that administration and staff don't understand Matthew's temperament, illness and complexity, but it is our only real option right now.

Luke is now eight and remains sweet, loving and the most sensitive of all our children. His odd snorting and behaviors reached a climax when he was seven. He would lay awake at night crying that he couldn't fall asleep because he couldn't stop making noises, clearing his throat, and flexing certain muscles. "It's driving me crazy mommy/daddy, please make it stop or I'll die" he cried. The pediatrician was once again at a loss. He suggested we seek further help. Despite strong reluctance as "it will just mean more meds", Jack too agreed for Luke's sake it was time he was seen. So, off we went with our second son to the psychiatrist. The diagnosis was not a surprise, and in my heart I already knew it when she spoke the words "Tourette's syndrome" with Attention Deficit issues. Jack took it the hardest as it was the death of a dream about Luke's complete normalness. Medicating Luke had proven difficult, and we continued on that long journey with him. Medications designed to help attentional issue interact negatively with the Tourette's and exacerbate his tics. He remains impulsive and high energy, and has difficulty focusing and staying on task. He is receiving special education support at school. He has good peer relations, but tries to hide that he is very anxious and worried most of the time. He wakes up afraid during the night, and his fear ranges from valid to unrealistic, and his tics range from severe or mild, depending on the day. We do a lot of comforting and calming, and our goal is to have him feel as comfortable as he can in his own skin. He asked me recently, "Some day when I get to heaven, mommy, will all my tics be gone?" It is a comment like that that goes deep into a mother's heart.

Hope is now three. From when she was first born we saw signs that we dreaded but ignored. She was different than Matthew, but bore striking similarities in areas like sleep and disposition. She too wouldn't sleep through the night and gave up naps at a year old. (Jack and I often joke that we haven't really slept in nine years.) Her temperament is dramatic and intense. Her mood changes frequently, and, like Matthew, she is engaging and charming, talking to anyone who will listen. Her artistic ability is amazing, and she is fun, intelligent and loving, but can quickly turn fiercely angry. She stands out in a crowd as she shares Matthew's angelic blond hair and blue eyes. Confirmations of our worst fears materialized when at age two she began talking to "fake people" as she called them. By age three, the "people" began tormenting her and teasing her. She would rip out her hair in frustration screaming "They're driving me crazy!" She saw them everywhere. She would scream at them in a grocery store, in her room, or the car. She insisted we carry her and would not touch the floor because "people" were all over the ground. It was chilling as we would sit in the dim light at three in the morning, while she would stare wild eyed behind us at visions of things we couldn't see. We had suffered through night terrors with the boys, but this was different. She was awake, responsive, alert and terrified. Parent's strongest desires are to protect their child, and it is agonizing to not be able to climb into her head to make them go away. We procrastinated and put it off as long as possible, but ultimately felt we needed to intervene for her sake. The pediatrician spoke quietly as he mentioned the word psychosis and suggested once again, we seek outside help. Hope began seeing the psychiatrist when she was three. She remains high energy and has frequent mood changes, but her sleep patterns are improved and she still mentions the "fake people", but they don't seem to torment her. We remain hopeful as she has responded well to very small conservative measures so far.

Our psychiatrist remains easily accessible, returns calls promptly, and remembers small details. We believe she truly has our children's best interests at heart and we never have to wonder if she knows who we are when we call. So, as we said in the beginning, our three children under the age of nine are under psychiatric care. As we write our chronicle, Jack laughs that our story "could be a book by itself". I agree, and we think about what the account of our life will do. Will we want our children to read this when they get older, we wonder. "There are no answers – even we haven't figured anything out" Jack says. I agree, but respond that even if one parent finds comfort or identifies with our story, it's worth it. I think we have learned many lessons, which have shaped us into who we are, and what our children will become. We diligently try to never be ashamed of them or their story. We try to provide lots of life experience from raising chickens to teaching them what their medications are, and what they do. Ultimately, it is their illnesses, and we want to prepare them for life ahead as best we can. We still struggle between knowing the difference of what is age related behaviors versus manifestation of the illnesses. We are forced to frequently try to reconcile feelings of pity for our children mixed with anger over the illness at the same time.

We have had to make hard choices. Jack works over sixty hours a week, and in his heart desires to dedicate himself to our business full time. But, because of doctors and prescriptions that top $3,000 a month, he is tied to the City for the health benefits.

We are learning the art of forgiveness as we have suffered needless shame and embarrassment from insensitive, uncompassionate people. I think of the pharmacist, who quizzed me on the possible side effects of one particular medication for Matthew. When I responded I understood the potential side effects, he stared at me in horror and said "And you're still going to give it?" He refused to fill the prescription until he had spoken to the doctor several times. I left feeling belittled and humiliated. I used to say that I wish those people could be "blessed" with a special needs child, so they could learn a lesson in humility and sensitivity. I am ashamed now that I was sarcastic with those words because I realize our children truly are a blessing.

Our children have taught us to practice silence, when well meaning people ask if we have ever considered a more "natural approach" than meds. They had no idea of the pain we had endured or the struggle of the decisions we have had to make. I often bite my tongue rather than try to explain the hours I have spent researching vitamins and nutritional supplements, as well as the long list of dietary modifications, and homeopathic "cures" we have tried. It is often easier to smile than share, how we give the kids high grade Omega fish oil and complete multivitamins, or that we have long ago gone whole grain, sugar free and organic in our household.

The Lord has taught us lessons in grace and compassion. My heart is more able now to reach out without judgment when I see a mother struggling with a difficult child. God only knows, what difficulties or pain she may or may not be facing. Jack too is learning those lessons, and he has become a mentor in the school system. He tends to mentor children similar to our own. He admits that his experience with our kids and their disabilities have enabled him to be more understanding, tolerant, sympathetic and compassionate towards these children.

We have also had to become educators. Mental health carries a tremendous stigma. To most people it is elusive and mysterious, or even imaginary, yet it is no less of an illness than Diabetes or Multiple Sclerosis. Yet because you can't see it, it is easier somehow to dismiss. Our children are beautiful, and looking at them you don't see easily recognizable symptoms. Many times any behaviors are usually looked upon as being spoiled or lack of parental guidance. We try to emphasize to people, that it is no different than any other medical condition. To those people, who chastise us on our use of medication, we explain that just as it would be cruel to withhold insulin from a diabetic child, or as a parent gives acetaminophen when a child has a fever, we have come to view medications differently than we did before. Sure, there are days that we would like to take everything away to see what would happen. But as of now, like it or not, it is a part of our lives. Jack relates living with mental illness like living with cancer and the medications like chemotherapy. "Without the meds, you know you don't have a shot, so you poison your body to try to conquer the disease. That's how I feel sometimes, like we poison our kids with these medications to try to give them some quality of life and a chance at living. Even with the meds there's no guarantee....and who knows what the short term or long term side effects really are" he says.

We have also had to learn to deal with overwhelming guilt. Sometimes I think it may be the meds for nausea I took when I was pregnant, or the meds at delivery. Perhaps we shouldn't have let them watch videos intended to make babies smarter, or maybe the boys were born too close together. We worry that we didn't lavish enough attention or gave too much. Maybe we didn't pray hard enough, trust enough, or have enough faith. Perhaps it would be easier, if we knew we were at fault, at least then there would be someone to blame.

My mother words that "it's not supposed to be this hard" still echo through our daily life. Jack thinks our story is that we are doing the best we can do. He remains cynical, but we are unified in our approach. We have to be a team or be ripped apart. There is a strong bond that sometimes only forms through joint trials. We agree that a person can sympathize and try to understand, but can never truly relate unless they are living it. "I don't even try to explain it anymore" he says. "Even if I took the time, they would never get it anyway. It's like everything else; you have to live it to get it." Our marriage is stronger than ever and surprisingly so is my faith. After all, for me it's really all about the story of faith. "Now faith is being sure of what we hope for and certain of what we do not see." (Hebrews 11:1)1 I continue to study, hope for and firmly believe that whether we see it or not, the Lord is working His healing in our lives. I pray for wisdom for the doctors they see and the pharmacists who fill their prescriptions. We have found many people who support us, but also others who suggest more extreme reasons for our suffering. Often well meaning they do not embrace us, but rather tell us children are demon possessed, under a curse or worse, have just ignored us in an attempt to avoid the reality that sometimes God just chooses it is not the time to heal. I trust in the Lord yet they are the voices that haunt me when it's been a long day. It is in my heart as a mother though where God speaks to me. He quiets all those voices and whispers of another hidden reason. "God brings men into deep waters not to drown them, but to cleanse them." His greater purpose will be revealed in time.

I do know that our story has taught us to perhaps to listen more, judge less and just support others who are suffering, even when we may not have any answers. I recall when Matthew was young and I sat at the children's hospital waiting room with a woman, who reached out and shared her story. She had a daughter with hemophilia and her prognosis wasn't good. Her and her husband struggled with the knowledge that their other child might be left without a sibling, so they decided to have a third child. Now it was several years later, and her oldest daughter was getting treated for the severe hemophilia, and this third child, now two years old, was in chemotherapy for Leukemia. I wish now I had listened better and showed more compassion. Her story haunts me. Her suffering was beyond my understanding.

Our pictures still show a happy family who has tons of fun, laughs a lot, spend lots of time together, and make the best of every day. We almost appear normal. But then again, what is normal anyway? As the psychologist Alfred Alder said "The only normal people are the ones you don't know very well." Despite everything we have been through, are going through, and will experience, the only thing I am sure of is what the Lord has spoken in His Word: "Many are the plans in a man's heart, but it is the Lord's purpose that prevails" (Proverbs 19:21)

Dr.A: We inherit from our parents genes for the physical looks, temperament, intellectual capacity, and diseases as well. It is a well established fact, that many ailments run in the families, including asthma, diabetes, heart disease, to mention just a few. The same applies to psychiatric conditions and learning disabilities. The chromosomal characteristics of an individual brain are responsible for the brain formation, especially at the stages of early development. Still, inheriting the genes does not mean that the carrier of them would be doomed to develop this disease or condition. It would be more accurate to state that for the most part we are born with a predisposition for certain problems, or talents. People, who carry the genes for cancer, do not always develop the full blown malignancy. Obviously, in those cases forces of environment unbeknownst to us get into play, somehow "correcting" the inherited flaw. On the other hand, serious or lethal illness may afflict the body, not carrying any predisposing genes. So, we are dealing with a powerful and at the same time delicate balance between genetic scripts and the milieu, part of which is the biological environment we do not know much about, and part of it is the social and emotional surrounding. History is abundant with examples of people born with learning disabilities (Albert Einstein) or mental illness (Sir Winston Churchill), who became epitomes of success and fame. Multiple studies showed that children born into loving and caring families, and stimulating surroundings deal much better with any inherited learning problems. How about the interface between mental illness and family milieu?

Chapter 7
**My Journey With Tim or
When Time and Love Is Not Enough**

Mrs. Hamilton: My story is about my struggles with parenting and caring for a child with severe mental illness. I had adopted my son Tim when he was twenty seven months old from Romania. My husband and I were first time parents in our late thirties. After unsuccessful infertility treatment, and a long and painful adoption process, we happily took home our new son, our forever child. We were so excited and relieved to finally become parents. We totally immersed ourselves in parenting and raising this little boy, we wanted to give him the world. I always told my son, when he asked why we adopted him: you were a little boy who needed parents, and we were parents who needed a little boy. It was a perfect fit we found each other. We always understood a child adopted from Eastern Europe could have health issues that may not be seen right away. These children are almost always developmentally delayed due to their orphanage living conditions we as Americans can only guess at. I was a nurse with years of critical care experience, and my husband also had a medical background in nuclear medicine. We felt prepared to get our son extra help and have him tested, so we could get him whatever services he needed. I thought and believed love and time would solve the worst of this child's needs and issues. What I still remember is how unprepared we were for this child's emotional needs. He did not understand the language, and communication was often frustrating for all three of us, but he picked up the language fast, just words at first but slowly we started to understand each other. Tim was a very tactile child: he touched everything just for sensation, and it was quite some doing getting him used to taking a bath in a tub, he did not like the feel of new clothes on his skin, or socks and shoes on his feet. Tim was difficult to feed; he only liked soft foods, no texture, mostly dairy and canned fruit. He would eat the same thing day after day. He was in a constant state of motion and never stopped. I swore he ever ran in his sleep. He also had very bad motion sickness, constantly throwing up after a few minutes of riding in the car. Everything scared him; he never wanted to be separated from us, not even in the same room. He often held on to our clothing as we walked around the house. He would pull us by our finger to be with or follow him; just being in eye contact was not enough for Tim. The worst was at night, bedtime and sleeping. He did not like to be alone in his room, and did not fall asleep easily. If it was a bad night, it would take me up to three hours to settle him down, so I could crawl out of the room an inch at a time and close the door. Tim frequently woke crying, his face soaked with tears and shaking the crib in panic, so I would have to start the bedtime ritual over. What really bothered me was his refusal to let us comfort him: he wanted us there and to be held, but it did not seem to calm or reassure him. It was so frustrating, but the only advice we were given was to let him cry, and be patient, and wait, "he has been through a lot." No matter what anyone said, I just couldn't' let him cry alone. Tim looked and sounded terrified; I really believed he was having nightmares, not temper tantrums, like everyone told me, and that I was just spoiling him. I was like the mother of a young infant waiting for the baby to sleep through the night. I was exhausted and feeling like a lousy mother, because I could not comfort my long awaited child, he would not bond with me. I was so jealous of his foster mother, who told me he was easy to feed, and ate everything she gave to her family, and he fell asleep around nine until when she woke him up in the morning after her kids went to school. What kind of magic did she have that I didn't? All I ever heard at the adoption agency support groups were the wonderful stories and happy families. I did not feel happy or wonderful; I wondered if I belonged on the island of misfit mothers? Eventually and slowly things changed for us; in several months I saw first hope of change. Tim woke up screaming one morning, but this time he was calling for mama, and when I went to get him he had his arms outreaching for me. I picked him up, and for the very first time Tim snuggled his head into my neck and signed in relief stopping crying. This was the sign I was hoping for: he was ready and able to bond, and maybe I wasn't a horrible non-magical creature, I had the mommy magic, I was "Tim's mother". It was not until years later I learned my sad feeling were possibly due to post adoptions depression, similar to postpartum depression. Adoptive parent's worst fear is the words "reactive attachment disorder." I did not want to think that's why Tim couldn't bond right away, and again the mantra "time and love" is what Tim needs. Services like speech, physical and occupational therapy were required to treat his developmental delays, and we started out with Birth-to-Three services when he was thirty-months-old. I have nothing but praise for their wonderful services from the state of Connecticut: they seemed to really understand Tim's situation. They provided extensive testing and good service plan, including at home speech, OT (occupational therapy), and PT (physical therapy), and a community based sensory group/OT play group. At that time Tim was said to be fifteen months delayed in all areas of growth and development. He also had sensory integration issues due to the lack of stimulation in his former orphanage environment. We noticed that Tim always had the downward tilt of his head when walking and playing. The OT specialist found that Tim was moving his eyes in the wrong direction. Next came a Pediatric eye surgeon consult, who diagnosed Exotropia caused by weak eye muscles (a form of strabismus). The weaken eye muscles did not allow his eyes to focus or work together. He was tilting his head down in order to have his vision clear and his eyes focus together. This eye condition could only be corrected surgically, which is what we did. Only years later I would read an article from a John Hopkins University study that linked Exotropia in children with mental illness comorbidity. The study showed a high percentage of children with Exotropia developing severe mental illness by adulthood.

After Tim turned three, Birth-to-Three tried to find similar services in our town. It turned out that when a child turns three, services are provided only for the school year, and may be extended for a month longer, if they have summer program. We found out that in order to continue OT we had to pick up the cost, because developmental delays were not a diagnosis covered under our private insurance. We appealed and were denied; paying for two summers out of pocket for Tim's OT he needed so badly. We learned early: if you want the best care you spend the money. Our thought was that it's better for him than paying for soccer; he really needed our "time and love." Tim was doing very well in a special education preschool program. The staff and the teacher were outstanding and supportive. Tim still remained delayed, but was catching up fast, although his high energy and limited attention span continued to be a daily struggle in school and at home. By the end of his second year with us Tim developed a wonderful personality; he smiled and laughed all the time. He enjoyed any new experience we could provide for him: zoo's, hiking, biking, swimming, hands on projects like arts and crafts, soccer and baseball. As long as he was busy and doing something physical he was happy and so were we. We wondered if he had ADHD because of never ending energy and short attention span, but were told it was too early for testing, and we should wait, because he was smart and had caught up more than anyone anticipated. Tim met his grade level requirement and could be moved to mainstream kindergarten.

Everyone kept telling us what a wonderful parents we were to have gotten Tim all the help he needed in order to succeed as well as he had. One statement which bothered me the most was: what a good thing we did adopting a child with so many needs. We did not intend to adopt a special needs child; it was like saying that you intended to give birth to a special needs child. We did not choose adoption for humanitarian reasons, we just wanted to be parents, have a family and share our love like everyone else. I never felt we did so much extra because he was adopted. We just did what I thought any parent should do, when the child has needs, not just special needs. We were doing what parents should do, their best job possible for the child's future, and I still believe it now.

By the end of his second year home we made the decision to adopt another child – a sibling for Tim, because he was doing so well: we loved being parents and having a family. It turned out that this would be another long process, even longer than it was to get Tim. Many things have changed in the adoptions arena, domestic and international; it became be a long wait.

Tim started kindergarten like any other five-year-old, buying a big boy book bag and going to the welcome school picnic at the beginning of the year. We toured his classroom and met his teacher, who was young, energetic and had experience with special education students. I thought it was too good to be true: little did I know that this was to be Tim's last good year at school for a long time. It did not take long for Tim's hyperactive and impulsive behavior to be seen as an issue in classroom. Despite his teacher's help, Tim's work was subpar and messy, with a daily struggle, and frustration. He did not understand why he had to stay still and do this boring school work with no wiggling, talking and walking around at will. It was pretty clear at this point Tim needed an evaluation for ADHD, but, as we learned, it could be done only when parents call for PPT. Then the recommendation could be made for an assessment. We were starting to learn that if you want something bad enough from the school – call for PPT! The evaluation was done by the school psychologist; Tim was very high on ADHD scale, impulsive and having almost nonexistent attention span. We needed more help. Next you have to go to the pediatrician with the evaluation in hand and discuss medications as treatment. Not every Pedi doc is in favor of it, so often you are left with more questions than answers. Do you continue to hope that behavior modification would work or are medications the next step? Even most of the literature is ambiguous on the subject. We decided to get an appointment with a child psychiatrist; being a nurse I still believe in an MD evaluation. Many pediatricians would order a medication for a child to avoid the stigma of a mental health label, which, I believe, is done for the parents and not for the child. A psychiatrist can answer your questions and has a full understanding of all of the medication options, which are many. It is also good to let the school know you are starting or changing a medication. The teachers tended to work with us better, when they understand a treatment plan is in place, and is managed by the doctor. We also found it valuable to have the school place our child on a daily written behavior chart, which is sent home with your child and helps tracking good and bad days. It also becomes a good tool to help the doctor regulate the medication dosage more accurately. It can help to determine trigger situations, or the time of the day, when medications could be wearing off. There is also an issue of trying different medications. Some of them have side effects or just do not work with your child's type of ADHD or physiology: this is why psychiatrists are better equipped to deal with these medications than pediatricians. Midway through the year we consulted with a child psychiatrist and started Tim on Adderall. It took a month to find the right dose, but it did seem to help with the school work and classroom behaviors. We also started medications for sleep, as our psychiatrist believed, that the disrupted sleep pattern could be contributing to Tim's behaviors. I was relieved, that someone understood our problems and didn't assign blame on poor parenting. In the end of the year Tim was on track for first grade, but was recommended for a summer school to keep up his reading and math skills. Little did we know that this year with his wonderful child psychiatrist was going to be Tim's last good year at school for a very long time, may be ever.

Our second adoption was going horribly wrong. We hoped to adopt from Romania again and take Tim with us for the cultural experience. We got a referral for a thirty- months-old boy, but were unable to get a visa from Romania, which at that time was under consideration to join the European Union and could not use adoptions of orphans to foreign countries. We even had our CT state senator and the US diplomat in Romania trying to help us and other families in a similar situation. After a year and a half the US State Department informed us, that Romanian government was denying any foreign adoptions indefinitely. So we started the process over again, this time in Moldova, a former breakaway province of Romania. The process seemed shorter, but the Moldovan adoptions system was fragmented at best. There was much repeated paper work, and everything needed state or federal seals. We lost our first referral due to an orphanage paper work mistake. It was months with the picture of the baby on the refrigerator, who never came home. While all this was going on, Tim started regular first grade without any additional services. As good as Tim was doing through the summer, it took him only one day at school for his impulsive and willful behavior to show up. This was the start of Tim's long and rocky school years, when nothing was ever easy, and every aspect of his school day came at a conflict. If it was not for messy work or constantly asking the teacher for directions, it was about his behaviors, or arguing, or defiance to follow rules. Tim became grandiose in his behaviors: took two rings from my jewelry box to marry another first grade girl. At home he felt he should handle his own affairs and did not need parents to tell him what to do or what was important. We spent several PPTs on just behavioral plans. Tim started getting more anxious, when the travel to get our second child got closer. He did not want to go with us, and, when it came down to buying his tickets, he just told us "I am not going there." So we ended up making arrangements for my sister to stay with Tim, and he seemed very relieved. We felt bad, that he did not want to travel with us and have this cultural experience. We brought our twenty-months-old daughter Sara home in the end of October, and to our surprise Tim really took to her and couldn't wait to show everyone his new baby sister. We did not have a lot of sibling rivalry, but he did act like the third parent and insisted he remembered his native Romanian language and could interpret what Sara was saying. We had chosen to use baby sign language as a way to decrease the communication frustration, and Tim took that over and developed his own form of signing to Sara. It became a real control issue for him. By late November everything with Tim was on a downward spiral, he was ether irritable and having temper tantrums, or crying and hanging on to us, stating that he was bored and had nothing to do, or he did not want to go to bed, because he was afraid of seeing things or nightmares. We tried to put him in an instructional soccer league, but it was a disaster. He was so aggressive, that it turned out to be a kick and spit session. School was also a strain on everyone; his behavior has been out of control. On some days he was constantly talking, not following directions, homework being a nightmare of crying and ripping up assignments. His psychiatrist felt that Tim was suffering from a mood disorder, and we should start mood stabilizers and antipsychotic medications right away. Tim was showing more psychotic symptoms, hearing and seeing things that were either distracting him, or scaring him and controlling his behaviors. We were floored, it was a surreal diagnosis to be given to any six -year -old, but I knew that our psychiatrist was right: Tim's mood and behavior were so out of the normal! I was scared for Tim: what kind of life was he going to have after being diagnosed so young? I did not have any exposure to pediatric psychiatry in nursing school; I did not know what would happen to his developing brain, if we choose the big gun medications now. We had to trust our psychiatrist that Tim would not get better on his own and may continue to get worse, his complete and long lasting mental health being at stake. Tim was suffering mental pain and we had to act fast! I pulled myself together and said a little prayer to God: help me so I can help my son! I would say this prayer mantra many times to God and myself over next few years. We started Tim on the medication that he would need for the rest of his life. I had to put him in the same category as a patient with a diagnosis of diabetes in need of insulin to be stable. The only thing harder than starting this medication is choosing people you can trust to with such personal information. I was not ashamed; I was worried for Tim and did not want him to be judged because of his diagnosis and the medications he was taking. The reaction we got from the family was very mixed – a few people understood our difficult situation, most felt it was too drastic of a move to make, we were jumping the gun, and he needed stricter parenting, military or parochial school. I even had someone telling me that they had friends in a similar situation with a child they just adopted, but they decided it was too much for their family to handle and surrendered their parental rights to the state. I spent a lot of time explaining that Tim had a medical diagnosis that needed treatment, not a finger pointing, or blaming, he was not a defective child with a lack of parenting. This explanation was going to be my repeated message and public announcement forever. I did get a lot of support from my fellow nurses and coworkers, they have been my saving grace and safe place to go and unburden myself. I had to say to myself many times, that my child needed me and I could do this, it is what moms do!

Meanwhile Tim did not do well on medications, developing nausea and vomiting, losing weight, or becoming drowsy, dizzy and emotionally flat. At school he at times had slurred speech, was falling asleep at his desk, and falling out of his chair. Our pediatrician felt that Tim was treated too aggressively, and our psychiatrist changed the treatment plan, but reiterated that Tim needed stronger medications because his symptoms and condition were severe. We quickly learned that there may be many medication changes to come, because there was no way to predict how Tim's physiology would react to any particular mediation, other than trial and error. Despite the medication changes, Tim's mood was worse, and he was either crying, or sleepy, with no relief. One day, after two straight hours of crying and Tim yelling at us that we need to make him better, we decided to admit him to the private hospital where his psychiatrist was on staff. It was the longest hour ride I ever had in my life: I kept questioning if was I doing the right thing? I was new to the psychiatric hospital scene, I felt like I was giving up on Tim and abandoning him to an orphanage all over again, would he ever forgive me? Tim stayed in the hospital for six days and was released being calmer and relaxed. He went back to school, and new meds seemed to work for about a month. We ended up in the same situation again: Tim was irritable, anxious, moody, and hostile towards anyone he thought was a perceived threat either at school or at home. We were constantly walking on egg shells surrounded by land mines just to avoid any blow ups that could lead to endless crying, hitting or property destruction. He stopped sleeping and started seeing spiders crawling on the walls and the window curtains; saw faces talking to him, was walking around with his hand in front of him in order not to see dark shadows, or hear people always wailing to scare, or hurt him.

We had to admit him to a different hospital, where the doctor felt that Tim was suffering from a form of autism called pervasive developmental disorder (PDD), because he was behind develop-mentally especially in his language skills. I was just dumb founded by this diagnosis, now I couldn't sleep – it was impossible that something so big could be missed by a team of multispecialty providers, working with Tim over the years! To me he had all the symptoms – manic to depressed fitting into the diagnosis of bipolar disorder. I was on a huge fact finding mission to understand about PDD/autism, its symptoms and presentation in children. One night I was up watching a special TV program about autism. I taped the program, and while watching it and seeing the children with early autism, I understood that they were not Tim: he had nothing in common with them. I confronted the doctor at the hospital and in my firm nurse tone told that I was Tim's mother and Tim's expert and insisted on discharging Tim to our regular psychiatrist. The doctor told me that I was still in shock from his diagnosis and needed to refer to DSM IV psychiatric coding book to confirm his expert diagnosis. A few decades in critical care nursing make you a quick thinker: I requested to discharge Tim to a Day Hospital Program, where he would be supervised by our psychiatrist. The hospital psychiatrist had to agree. I am still not sure what that doctor motives were, but pretty convinced it had to do with me challenging his diagnosis (his ego). I felt Tim needed to come home and be with his family, with his mom, not the institutional caregiver; he has had enough of those in his young life already! We did our first of many intakes, which is an interviewing and screening process to evaluate if someone is a good candidate and would benefit from the program. It really hit me hard that Tim was so ill and had become so dysfunctional at home and school, that we were now talking about his entire future on medications and fighting for his mental stability. I was afraid to think how deep did this go? Is every aspect of Tim's life is going to be dependent on medical management of his mental illness? The answer I have come to know and live with deep in the heart is YES! He will never again be just Tim, he will forever be a person with a lifelong chronic illness, and he will always have an uphill battle to fight for his mental wellness. Tim was admitted to the partial hospital program, maintaining the schedule of ½ day school and ½ day treatment, including medication management, groups and individual therapy. Tim's teacher and I were getting concerned about the amount of school he was missing, because he was starting to fall behind, and his grades were suffering. All doctors told me to worry about his mental health first; his school work can be made up. The day hospital program was intense, but it was slowly working. We went to all family nights and parent counseling, spoke with the doctors every few days and tried many different medications. Tim was a difficult child to medicate because he seemed to have all bad and rare reactions, and not a lot of benefits. ADHD medications could cause mania in many people with bipolar disorder; we also saw antidepressants caused mania with Tim. He was a mixed bag of symptoms and problems. His RAD diagnosis had become a reality to us and the explanation of some of his disruptive behaviors, including stealing, defiance and mistrust. This was such a long process for me. I have been a surgical and critical care nurse most of my career, used to quick diagnosis and treatment, weighing quick results. Mental health diagnosis and treatment for me seemed to take an eternity with minimal results over long periods of time. I am better at accepting this now, but it is still hard to watch someone suffer and hope it may work out, maybe someday.

As Tim was finishing his school year he had his final planning PPT. I felt he needed to stay back a year, or be put in a special education classroom or program. I did not get very far: Tim was allowed to have only some extra help, and not considered in need of special education services, because I was doing such a good job taking care of his mental health needs. They felt he could be caught up in summer school. Again I tried to remind them that his current mental stability may go away at any time, and his medications can make him sleepy and forgetful, and cause him problems with retention of information. No one wanted to hear me. As I learned later, the school system does anything they can to avoid paying for expensive special education services and teachers. Tim's mental illness was not going to be recognized as a disability to his learning, because he had an average to high IQ score. We got through summer school in July and did swim and tennis lessons. In august many things fell apart and Tim became manic, moody and irritable. My husband was the primary caregiver at home, because my full time job carried the best health benefits. And Tim needed constant supervision, and there was not a day care provider who would take a child with a severe mood disorder on the amount of medications Tim took. I do not know if it was the stress or the fear of having a child with a mood disorder, but my husband and Tim were always at odds. Their constant bickering was disruptive to the house, and now my husband started to blame me that I was not letting the doctor know how bad Tim's behavior was. I couldn't get my husband to understand, that a child's bipolar disorder can be just as devastating as an adult, because they do not have many coping skills yet, and do not understand what is going on in their brain – it is just beyond a child's cognitive ability. And I reminded him that when he was diagnosed with Bipolar Disorder in his twenties, he was unable to work or go to school. Most adult are completely incapacitated with this disease, but we expect children to continue to function on the same level they were before they got sick, and succeed in school. We had made several medication changes over the summer, but Tim was barely functioning by the start of school in September. By the second week of school during open house I could see Tim couldn't even sit in a chair and follow simple directions without becoming frustrated or confused. Shortly after Tim became angry and moody, talking back or laughing inappropriately and sometimes downright rude. It only took a week or two, and Tim was back in the hospital with raging mania. A new round of medications to try, hoping to get some stability back. The next blow came, when we found that our psychiatrist was leaving his private practice, and would be only practicing in the inpatient hospital. This meant we had to find another doctor. We had made many phone calls only to find out, how few child psychiatrists are there and how even fewer were taking new patients. And Tim's case was so complicated by his multiple diagnoses; I think we intimidated a few docs just during the intake appointments. We interviewed with the psychiatrist our previous psychiatrist recommended. She had unflustered acceptance of Tim's multiple diagnoses, and understood what having RAD meant for an adopted child from an eastern European orphanage. During the first interview she couldn't believe that we have been able to care for Tim at home with no extra services. Right away she suggested neurocognitive testing either through the school, or our insurance, to get him into full time special education classroom or a private special education school: he was too disabled to continue mainstream. It took full eight weeks to find someone at the children's hospital and get the insurance approval, because the school still did not feel Tim needed full time special education. The testing took two days instead of one, because after the first evaluation it was clear that Tim needed extra services. His ADHD was off the scale, he showed cognitive delays, and his mood disorder was delaying and impeding his learning. Of course, everything at school was going downhill: no work getting done along with constant disruptions in the classroom due to his impulsive and inappropriate behaviors. At one low point Tim's teacher was so frustrated with Tim making rude comments and gestures to him, that he stuck his fingers in his own ears. Tim responded with: "Bring it on, BALDIE!"- putting him into a well deserved and needed suspension for that day. The next few weeks were just constant phone calls from the school regarding Tim's behavior or lack of such. I finally gave up in tears and told the vice principle to do whatever he wanted to, suspend Tim, call DCF, call for emergency PPT. I was just a mom with a sick child, and a pending neuropsychiatric evaluation, so I could get him into special education program. I stated I had done everything I could, he was on medications, had been hospitalized, under doctor's care and if the school could not help me then I would keep Tim home, and they could send a tutor with military training to our home, and I would just retain an attorney until someone listened to me. The vice principal was quiet for a long pause and then stated, that he did not realize how serious the situation was, and would personally get the ball rolling with the board and referral for special education. For the first time in months I felt relief, but it was short lived: Tim went into a total rage that weekend, became manic and was admitted again. We had our final PPT in public school while Tim still was in the hospital. The head of the department of special education school board lead the meeting. She started with the statement, that Tim's evaluation had eighteen special need provisions the public school was unable to meet. With his level of severe disabilities he would immediately be outsourced to a private special education school that had an opening for a new student. This was a very hard fight for the victory, but not our last battle as we were to find out. We were interviewed a couple of days later at a clinical day school. We took Tim on a day pass from the hospital with us. His affect was so flat and he was so unemotional from all the meds that he did not seem to understand what was going on. He was just glad to be out of his old school, because he was not happy there and frustrated most of the time. We also decided to accept DCF voluntary services and request in home family therapy. This program would include 2-3 times a week visits from two therapists to work with us and Tim, to develop better parenting strategies, and to decompress the stress at home. Tim and my husband still had daily conflicts, and Tim's constant demand for attention was draining us all. Tim seemed to adjust slowly to his new school setting; he honeymooned with good behavior for a few weeks, and then started acting up on a daily basis, refusing to do his school work. He was still struggling with mood stabilization, and his psychiatrist and I tried several different medications and dosages with short term effect. But we did notice a pattern with Tim's behaviors and started to suspect a seasonal element: depressed and moody in the winter changing to manic and irritable in the spring. Things were improving at home with Tim less oppositional and more following directions. But school was still a problem: the principal, therapist and the school psychiatrist had called us for PPT to discuss his lack of educational progress and lack of cooperation with assignments. I was wondering, if he was not doing the work because he did not understand it: he had missed so much school in the past year being in the hospital or listless. With all the medications changes he was just too far behind to catch up and needed to be placed in a lower functioning group. I felt ridiculous to remind them, that Tim had huge gaps in his education over the past two years, and frustration might account for some of his behaviors. He has simply given up; the work was too hard for him. What really was happening – the school wanted to re-label his mood disorder diagnosis to autism/mental retardation because of his flat affect, and lack of cooperation, and progress in school. I stated Tim was not always like this before he got sick; he was a happy kid who laughed, got excited at new things, he had a full range of emotions, and had met his developmental milestones. And he learned English as a second language, had high verbal skills and was on track educationally, until mid way through first grade. I refused to accept this diagnosis in the past, as it did not fit him, and I was still refusing to allow it. Now the school psychiatrist spoke, and I found out he was

Romanian. He asked where did we adopt Tim from, and I said your native country of Romania. He seemed a little perturbed by that, and then he asked what part of Romania, and I knew where this was going. I stated Bihor County. And he asked where in Bihor, and I reluctantly said Solanta (it is a northern village in the Carpathian Mountains, with a large Romani populations). As I have seen firsthand and was told by our adoption agency, many Europeans are prejudiced against house of Romani (gypsy) heritage and consider them third class citizens, not deserving basic human rights. He replied that it was a very poor area with a lot of abandoned children, no prenatal care and large orphanages. Tim could have some brain damage, and mental retardation could be his problem. I stated that this diagnosis was brought up by Tim's doctors, only when they got frustrated trying to medicate his resistant mood disorder. When he and the therapist asked why I was so against this diagnosis, I explained that I knew Tim before getting sick, I stayed in contact with his teachers from that time, and they did not believe it either. But most importantly, our psychiatrist and I know he is intelligent, and, as she has told me many times, a child with this illness has inaccessible intelligence until he is well enough to show it. By now PPT just turned unproductive and our special education counselor from our home school (whom I did not know well then, but who would come to be a great ally of ours) asked: "What are we going to do to move forward with his education, and isn't it time to make a plan for summer school if Tim is so far behind?" The principal reluctantly agreed to place Tim in a lower functioning classroom for the reminder of the school year. But Tim was too demanding to have in their summer program; they only took high functioning students. I was totally confused and said: "So you are in alleged special education school, but only for good kids, not the ones who need it the most?" The therapist felt it would be best for us to look for other summer school programs, and let them know how he did, before coming back in the fall. The school board counselor, Tim's ICAP advisor, and I met outside and agreed we were just given the boot, and the ball was in our court now. I interviewed three school programs for developmentally delayed children. The first one wondered why we were there; Tim was too high functioning for them. The second was mostly for residential students, and we were not at that point yet. The third was a special education school with a good reputation and far from our home town, but the facilities were beautiful, brand new, and they seemed positive that they could handle Tim and his needs. We enrolled him in their six week summer program. By then Tim finished his school year, and I called the principal to let them know, that we found a summer program, and I also inquired how Tim was doing in his new class. The principal had to admit that he was doing better with his behaviors and doing his classroom work again. We decided Tim would not be returning there in the fall. Tim was in a stable period that summer and did very well in the new summer program. I think he was relieved to be there: they had fun classes, he was outside a lot, and they had a pool on the grounds. The school started off all right, but soon deteriorated, as his mood started changing again. We had conflicts on the bus; he got bored with the long rides, did not want to do therapy groups, and was too irritable. Things were also difficult at home – he was always pushing his limits and boundaries at home with his father. There were battles over the house rules and broken items after his fits and rages. I never knew what was coming at me when I came home. Again, we tried many medication changes, and Tim still ended up in the hospital with rapid cycling of his moods. The school seemed totally confounded by Tim's behavior. I got the feeling they did not believe or understand a true bipolar child and that he was very sick. It just was a constant conversation about him not responding to the behavior protocols and still raging. We acquitted the services of an educational advocate to help us to deal with the school and the board of education. We were at odds with everyone; it was like the school had never had a child like Tim. They were shocked and surprised every time Tim had a behavioral problem. We kept changing his medications, and at one point the school contacted our psychiatrist because they did not believe that Tim was in treatment, and thought we were just bad parents allowing the child to act this way because of the care he got at home. Our psychiatrist set them straight and informed them, that we were good parents doing our best to take care of a very sick child, who would be living in a long term hospital without us. And she was not surprised by his behaviors: Tim had a mood disorder and could have psychotic and depressive episodes with little warning. The worst was during one of Tim's rages: he ran out of school, down the street and was throwing rocks at the cars. The school was able to get him back on the grounds, but as soon as his classroom aide turned her back on him (which one should never do), he threw a rock at her and caused a bruise on her shoulder. The school pressed charges, and Tim was arrested when he was eight years old, being released to my custody, provided I take him to the hospital for an evaluation. Completely stunned by the school pressing charges we decided to admit him for observation and to protect him from further prosecution. I hired a family law attorney, who could not understand why a special education school would press charges on a child under their care with known mental illness! He was very reassuring to me that this would not go far in criminal court, because Tim was already getting services for his condition and this was an isolated episode. But he also warned me that the staff person at his school could take this to civil court and sue us. After a few sleepless nights it ended quickly, when the local police dropped the charges, because Tim was only eight, and as the court officer said: "He did a bad boy thing not something criminal, and she wished the school would stop calling them and handle their own problems." We decided to deescalate the situation by placing him back in a partial day hospital program for the rest of the year. It was ironic, that we had to do this, after Tim supposedly was already in a therapeutic psychiatric setting. After this incident we had our end of the year PPT, where I brought my team of providers, and the school brought in everyone except for the janitor for their side. That was one of my top three worst PPTs. The school would not back down on their position, stating that they had done everything they could for Tim and were not making any adjustment to his IEP. That's when I found out from his therapist, that Tim had not been seen by her since December because they did not connect well. I was outraged that the eight- year- old got to decide his treatment plan, and was wondering why they called them "special education" when nothing special was going on. They insisted, that Tim was too demanding for their setting, and it was decided and agreed upon he could only stay if he had one to one support. Luckily the school board agreed, and extra help was given to the classroom just for Tim's needs. The writing was on the wall for us, and after Tim finished the summer program, we started looking for another school again. This school board advisor had given us the name of a different clinical day school. The intake went great: I was totally honest that we were there, because every other school claiming to be special education gave up on Tim. I made it clear, that Tim needed a school able to deal with his disabilities, and understand, that when his moods cycle, he may end up in the hospital, and the goal of the day would be just keeping him safe. They felt Tim was smart and that they could work with him. We started a few weeks later, and it took only a little time to understand, that Tim was far behind in education, missing a lot of the last few years to either illness absence or behavior. He was tested and found to have his IQ drop from 98 to 68 in two years. I felt it was not accurate, as in the literature children on heavy psychotropic medications like Tim often do not score well. We all felt it was in Tim's' best interest to continue in a lower skills class, and give him the time he needs to learn at his own pace and with a lot of extra help. Unfortunately Tim's mood disorder got the better of his first year: he was unstable with frequent visits to the hospital. We ended up this year only on a half day at school, because it was all Tim could handle. There have been a lot of PPTs and planning since Tim's first year at this school, we have all learned from each other and Tim over the last three years. There have been quite a few rough patches and changes to his program, and more than one uncomfortable PPT regarding Tim's outrageous behaviors. But we have learned to trust and listen to each other, and bounce ideas around, understand, and most importantly accept Tim's limits. He is a very sick child, with his illness at times becoming totally debilitating. But the school stuck it out with Tim, and there were a few times I honestly couldn't believe they kept him at school. There was a time recently, when Tim was so manic at school and at home, that we actually interviewed with the state DCF to possible get him admitted to a long term care hospital. We had to admit him to the only hospital, where the bed was available, and where I had an argument with the attending that did not recognize the bipolar disorder in Tim. Here we were again: the doctor and the therapist said Tim was acting out because of his RAD diagnosis, and he was not getting the right therapy. They did not recognize the seasonal component and felt, that he had PTSD, and must have had a bad experience during the winter, and got depressed. To which I said: "From what I know firsthand of eastern European orphanages it SUCKED there all the time and I bet there wasn't just one time you could pick out over the rest!" He basically thought we all did not know what we were doing and had it all wrong. I wanted to know, why he thought after all this time and hard work we have put into Tim, he was the only right opinion. He stated: "Well, I have been to medical school, not you!" I replied again: "I'm Tim's expert, not you, and a nurse, working with hundreds of doctors over the last twenty eight years. Going to medical school isn't all that, and if that's all you have to back up your theory, I want Tim discharged!" Well, another bridge burned under my belt, but sometimes you have to go with what you know works. Our doctor, me, and the school went back to the drawing board and started over again. We ended up admitting Tim back to the hospital again two months later in a mixed manic and depressed state. For the first time Tim actually told me he wished he were dead and not feeling the way he did anymore. We had to take drastic steps: it was decided we should do a medication washout and start Tim on Clozaril. We had tried over thirty five medications in the last four and half years with only short periods of stability, and Tim was turning twelve, and starting puberty soon, and surge of hormones could make him even worse than now. It was one of the most terrible hospitalizations: he looked so sick and felt miserable. We had to consult with a hematologist, because his white blood count was low from years of being on Seroquel. Clozaril is a serious medication for adults to start, and not many children are on it, only the sickest and we were there! We had to place him in a national registry per FDA rules because of the potential lethal side effects. I was just nauseous over the idea but felt it was our last line of treatment, or Tim may become so unstable, that he could not live at home ever again. As one of our doctor's patient's parents said: you have to look at this as if it were chemotherapy. We started, and over the next few weeks and months Tim improved, and we continued treatment. It has been rough dealing with frequent blood draws, and the FDA registrant guideline, but it has been worth it to see the change in Tim. I have noticed, the school has noticed, and Tim was brought himself up to a grade level. We also have started Lithium to help with the mood stabilization and increase his white blood count, at times dropping dangerously low, so he can continue taking the Clozaril. This medication has changed Tim's life for the better, but he still had a lot of work to do to catch up with his age group. It was so pleasant, going to PPT when Tim did well, and the teachers were pleased and proud of his progress. We all hoped and prayed it continues. I'm like any other parent – I just want the best. I try to keep an open mind about medications, treatment options, and try to keep up on the few reputable medical websites for any new studies or findings. Keeping informed has only helped me and my son, not settling for less, when there can be more to try. This not a cure, but a milestone for us, a possible way to keep his moods stable for longer periods of time. Having a child that ill completely changes your life in a way you may not be prepared for. The relationship between my husband and son has deteriorated over the years to just animosity: like a big brother and a little brother they argue about everything and want me to solve all their problems, placing the blame on each other. They call 911 on each other as a threat, and have a hard time being civil to each other. This has taken its toll on our family, and our marriage, and my personal relationship with my husband. Tim's younger sister will grow up with a brother with severe mental illness, witnessing all the horror that comes with that. We have support for her, and just recently I placed her in an after school program, so she spends as little time with her brother and dad as possible. I have been trying to find an after school program that can accommodate Tim's needs, but did not have any luck yet; even in a therapeutic program he still is high maintenance. The possibility of Tim ending up in a residential care grows with each passing month, as he grows and may become too big or unsafe for us to care for him at home. It kills me to think I may have to give up my long awaited forever child to accept he is more than I can handle. There is no magic or cure – only lots of tears, frustration, stress, vigilance, constant care giving and ongoing fear, prejudice and worry for the parent of a mentally ill child. There is very little understanding and support for you and your child, you may and will lose your friends, family, marriages and care providers. Your struggle is not like with a physical illness. You will seldom get emotional support or good advice, and many times you or your child will be blamed for this illness and behaviors. There are very few who will understand or care to understand your situation. Almost no one will step forward to help out and give you a break. This is truly parenting on the edge, where surviving the day is the best you can do. Only a few people give me hope and support. I have come to rely on our psychiatrist and her words of advice and comfort, and frank honesty. She is willing to try and help Tim as long as she and I can do this; she has never given up or settled for less than the potential for a full life for Tim. Nothing is written in stone for her. I need and admire that quality, trust her judgment on what we can do, but most importantly what I can do as a mother with a sick child. She values my observations and opinions, we work great together and she helps me to accept the consequences and limitation of Tim's illness. I have my younger sister who completely accepts Tim and his illness, and my struggles and supports me without questions or limitations. She is my rock and my trustworthy person I do not have to make excuses to. When I told her the title of this story, she said I needed to call it a rescue mission, not just a journey. I have found support and friendship with Tim's teacher and therapist at his school and have become a charter member of the Parent and Faculty advisory board at his school; this has allowed me to meet with other parents and share wisdom and tears, and write a few articles for the school newsletter. I have also great support of my fellow nurses as they see my struggles and help to celebrate Tim's victories. There is always a kind word and a helping hand when I feel defeated. I have my blessing and my struggles – it is just keeping it all in balance - that's difficult. Time and Love that's what I got.

Dr. A: This story is a book by itself. Let me address two aspects of it, and the rest I will defer to our panel for additional comments. The first is medical: the complexity and controversy of diagnoses and treatment of children psychiatric conditions. Tim had an insidious onset of his problems, which initially presented as "ADHD" and responded to ADHD designated medications for a while. What makes it difficult diagnostically - is the overlapping of some symptoms of ADHD and mood disorder, especially poor impulse control, shortened attention span, difficulties following directions and defiance. The early indication of possible mood disorder, overshadowed by the attentional issues, would be controlling and bossy behavior – quite grandiose for a small child. Most of the pediatricians are not ready to tease out one state from another, which is not their fault. They did not have appropriate training and even nowadays are not being educated about children mental illness. Even the psychiatrist, who dealt with Lynne twice in the hospital, insisted on RAD or autism, totally overlooking severe mood swings and psychotic symptoms. Just that part should have been enough to at least suspect, that this is "out of the box" child, showing more symptoms NOT fitting into a conventional diagnosis he had in mind, than consistent with his diagnostic mold. The system for the most part failed Lynne and Tim on several different levels, educational, medical, and behavioral. Children with mental illness are "homeless" educationally as well as medically. Lynne is a trained medical professional in one of the most dynamic and difficult medical specialties – critical care, used to quick thinking and feisty decisions. She understands MEDICINE. Imagine a parent in her shoes, who does not know anything about medications, or lab work, or cannot understand the medical jargon. The information becomes quite confusing causing parents feel lost between multiple, sometimes mutually antagonistic opinions. The problem lays in the lack of recognition of medically based child psychiatric conditions and lack of communication between providers. Quite commonly an attending physician in the hospital seeing a patient for the first time feels comfortable to make a totally different diagnostic determination without even contacting the outside providers. As a result, the whole treatment plan is being drastically changed, although the length of admission does not exceed several days, while it takes a long time for the body to respond and to adjust to every new medication change. Lynne presents as a model for all parents, insisting on what she believes is right for her child and putting herself in charge of the situation. I want to remind all parents that they are legal guardians of their children, and NOBODY can change any medications or use any treatment without their consent. Quite often I hear parents saying: "Medications were changed in the hospital and I do not think they work." To my question why they did not say "no" to the change I usually hear: "We did not know that we can say no!" Yes, you can, and you have to! Whenever we (adults) are recommended a new medication or treatment by our physicians, we usually either sign an informed consent, or get explanations why the recommended treatment may work. The same is true for our children; we need to know what they are taking, and what it may entail in a good or bad way. The educational and placement part is not less complicated. The schools and even the special education programs are not equipped to handle children like Tim. They are oriented toward children more amenable to behavioral interventions and less symptomatic than Tim. To begin with, special services or outplacements are expensive. Children who are bright, but have learning disabilities and psychiatric symptoms, like Anderson family children, or Tim fall through cracks. So far the parents are left to their own devices, going through the exhausting trial and error route in search of the best program to accommodate their children needs.

—————————————————————— Intermission ——————————————————————

Mrs. Anderson: I have found that neither medical nor educational systems are primed to deal with children with mental illness. As each child displays the symptoms in a wide variety of moods and behaviors, how can I expect to know for certain if this is the accurate diagnosis of my child?

Dr. A: You are correct. I'm afraid that differences in diagnostic approaches are quite common for medicine in general. In child psychiatry it is even more so, as it is a relatively "young" (no pun intended) discipline. Over the last decade the idea of children suffering from a psychiatric illness, as well as the adults, gradually penetrated into medical community, making at least some of the psychiatrists reconsider their diagnostic approaches. The public perception though still is encased into the old paradigm of poor parenting skills and family flaws causing child's problems. There is no perfect mental health picture, either for adults or children. To complicate things even more, as Mrs. Mertz indicated, mental illness is an "invisible" phenomenon; it is visible because of the behavioral, emotional or learning problems, but nobody can offer a blood test or an X-ray in order to show what's going wrong. Let me try to address your and other parents concerns regarding the discrepancy of the diagnoses. Many times over I heard from different parents: "How come that we saw so many psychiatrists and nobody told us that our child has a mood disorder?" We do not have any clear classification of childhood psychiatric conditions, except for very few, like Autism or ADHD. So, some labels from the adult classification migrated into the child nomenclature, creating a lot of confusion. You do not take your children to the adult department store to buy them clothing, toys and games, and even furniture; you take them to children's stores. But when it comes to psychiatry, we operate with adult terminology. One of the biggest misconceptions is the diagnosis of Bipolar Disorder (BD). About 12-15 years ago every single child I saw had been previously diagnosed with ADHD or Asperger's, which is a form of autism. Now almost all children come with the diagnosis of BD, which is an adult diagnosis and so far does not have a clear "child" version.

In order to be diagnosed with BD adults need to meet quite rigid criteria of severity and length of the symptoms: i.e. one or more manic or mixed (a combination of manic and depressive symptoms) episodes, at a minimum of one week duration, with or without history of depressive episodes. There are different subtypes of BD, with a different duration and severity of manic and depressive episodes. There is also a diagnosis of Cyclothymia, made when a patient has mild mood swings, not sufficiently severe to be diagnosed as mania or depression, and Dysthymia (sub-threshold depression lasting at least two years). There is also BD Not Otherwise Specified, when patients have manic and depressive symptoms not meeting the criteria for regular mania or depression. In order to be diagnosed with a depressive episode, patients would present with at last two weeks of depressed mood, or loss of interest or pleasure, along with changes of activity, sleep, energy level, lack of concentration, change of appetite and weight, suicidal thoughts or plan/attempts. Those symptoms would cause significant distress in all areas of patient's life, as well as functional impairment. A manic episode in adults presents with at least one week of expansive, elevated or irritable mood, with inflated self esteem or grandiosity, decreased need for sleep, distractibility, pressured speech and excessive talking, increased level of energy, disinhibited behavior, mostly aimed at having pleasurable experience as shopping, gambling, sexual escapades etc. It may seem obvious when people suffer from BD, but it still remains an elusive diagnosis, because of the increased incidence of sub-threshold mood phases and mixed episodes. The statistics of incidence of BD keeps changing. Comparing with schizophrenia, which is steadily diagnosed in 1% of the adult population throughout all countries and ethnicities, the incidence of BD fluctuates, depending on the diagnostic criteria, reaching up to 5% according to some sources. Approximately 69% of BD patients remain misdiagnosed, with about ten year gap between the onset of symptoms, and the correct diagnosis and appropriate treatment. The delay of the diagnosis and consequently appropriate interventions result in the increased cost of treatment (estimated at 24 billion in US in 1998 and rising), increased suicidal rate, chronic debilitating course with the decline of functioning and quality of life. The accurate estimate of BD is problematic due to the differences in opinions among adult psychiatrists (here comes the ten year gap before the correct diagnosis is made), and increased incidence of mixed forms which are difficult to recognize right away.

Obviously adult criteria do not fully apply to children. To begin with, children cannot maintain the same mood for the extended length of time as adults do, as their nervous system remains immature. I was recently watching a two- year- old child playing on the beach: he was going from desperate crying to a happy smile in a flash. One moment he fell and was inconsolable, but as soon as his father took him into his arms and showed him something interesting, the tears dried up and child was laughing. This is a totally normal child with the appropriate for his age range and volatility of his emotions. For a 5-6- year- old this emotional roller coaster would be concerning, but not qualifying him of her for the diagnosis of any mood disorder, just based on this presentation.

We are looking for correlates of mood instability in children. Very infrequently children before puberty would present with similar to adults manic symptoms. Only a few times I saw young children truly grandiose. For example, one of them stated he would enter any house and become an invisible spy; another one had "super vision" and assured me he was seeing many layers in the walls of my office, including molecular ones; another child used to come in a costume of a superman and attempted to show me how he flies etc. But mostly "manic" children present with arrogant, condescending attitude, coming across as if they are adults, talking as adults, giving their parents or their teachers at school directions how to do things, and not responding to any limit setting. They attempt to co-parent their younger siblings (as Tim took charges with his baby sister) demanding total obedience. It is not uncommon to hear from teachers, that the child states nobody can tell him/her what to do; they follow their own schedules, get out of their seats and walk out of the classroom disregarding any rules or regulations. Any power struggle or limit setting makes them furiously angry and even more confrontational. They usually get the diagnosis of Oppositional Defiant Disorder and do not respond to any punishment or boundaries setting. A while ago I coined the term "Oppositional Psychotic Disorder", more accurately describing the problem. This behavior is commonly mistaken for the personality or upbringing flaws, and believed to be handled with just appropriate behavioral modification plans, which expectedly fail. Behavioral plans are helpful, when the medical cause of the behavior is taken care of with medication, which frequently does not happen soon enough. Both depressed and manic children may present as irritable and angry. When depressed, they become sad and tearful, losing interest and drive, getting worse grades or even failing, becoming more isolative and withdrawn. Neither of those mood phases last for a long time; most of the children do not present with a one-dimensional emotional condition. Typically they have kaleidoscopic mood shifts, many times a day, or even an hour, going from being angry, irritable, to happy and giggly, clown-like, aggressive, to sullen, tearful and withdrawn, or mixed phases with some traits of depression and mania (the child version of both) at the same time. As you see, the "bipolar" term does not capture the complexity of the picture: children usually present with "multipolar" disorder. One six-year-old boy I evaluated at school drew a roller coaster on the chalk board and said: "This is me and my moods!" Older children, especially pre- and adolescents, when manic, would become preoccupied with sex, making lewd statements, or grabbing their peers, sometimes even teachers, talking about their sexual escapades never taking place. Most of those presentations evoke punitive steps at school; less often a psychiatric consult is requested.

So far we were talking about just mood changes and concomitant behavioral changes noticeable to any minimally astute observer. Not uncommonly they are only the tip of the iceberg: children, especially young, would experience psychotic symptoms, hearing voices inside and outside their head, seeing thing both inside and outside their actual field of vision, without telling anybody about their unusual experiences. Sometimes those visions become very complicated: quite a few times children described in details the world existing in their minds, sometimes made of glass or some unusual materials, inhabited with different creatures, at times scary and at times entertaining.

Mrs. Strom: Why do you think it is not just a fantasy world? Children are imaginative, they like to play and fantasize, and they have imaginary friends. Are you saying that any fantasy is a sign of a disease?

Dr. A: Of course, not. There is a difference between a fantasy and what's called impaired reality testing aka psychotic symptoms. The fantasy is always under control of its creator; he or she can always put it on hold and switch this imaginary world on and off. When the "fantasy" takes the life of its own, taking over the judgment, performance, actions, especially in a dangerous way, it becomes a disease. Psychotic voices (auditorial hallucinations) tell children and adults to do bad things, hurt themselves, run away, jump out of the window, and talk back. One of the children I recently evaluated was hearing voices of the monsters telling him: "Be bad! Hit! Run!" The same is true regarding traditional monsters under the bed. It is an expected fear for a young child, goes away with age, does not affect the daytime activity and can be handled with reassurance, favorite toys, dream catchers etc. The developmentally appropriate fear is an encapsulated phenomenon; impaired reality testing goes outside this "capsule" spreading onto the life and affecting it in a negative way. Let me give you an example of a paranoid perception. If we walk through dark, unsafe neighborhood, known for its high crime rate, we feel uncomfortable, but calm down as soon as we reach a well lit crowded street with a police car at the corner. If a person thinks that he/she is being followed no matter when and where he/she is going, that all cars in the street are following him/her, and video monitors are set in his/her apartment, we would rightfully suspect that this person suffers from paranoid ideation. If such thoughts affect the life to the extent, that this person stops leaving the apartment, does not go to work, stops sleeping, does not eat, and shows impairment in the usual level of functioning, it becomes quite clear, that the person needs medical help. Not all adults, who develop psychiatric problems, can articulate what is going on with them: only the changes of their behavior would suggest that something dire is taking place. Children, especially young ones, cannot be expected to explain that they are not "right"; we can only see their behavior changing. One of my adult patients asked me to see her five-year-old son. She was often complaining that he never mastered toilet training, despite many hours spent with different psychologists, multiple behavioral plans, reward system and other "tricks" she learned from other parents. Recently this child, who has always been bright and outspoken, started to misbehave at school, getting out of his seat, singing in the middle of the lesson, refusing to cooperate with the school rules, and not in the least being embarrassed with his "accidents". This little boy indeed turned out to be extremely eloquent and outspoken. When I asked him my favorite question "why", he immediately proceeded with the following story. In many details he described to me that for quite some time he saw aliens inhabitated the bathrooms and especially the toilet paper rolls. They surrounded him in any place and made him fearful to use the potty or the toilet. He went even further telling me about him swimming in the ocean far from the coast and getting away from sharks. I was listening to him for a long time: he had more fantastic stories to tell. When he talked about his adventures his face remained flat, he spoke in a monotone, without much of an inflection, in a rapid way, and could not stop. I asked his mother to join us, and requested that the child would repeat what he said to me. He willingly did so. The mother was shocked and attempted to "correct" the stories, reminding her son that he had never swam in the ocean alone, making him extremely angry with her comments. The mother became angry and hostile, when I attempted to explain to her the true reason for the failed toilet training: ongoing psychotic and hypomanic symptoms. This not an uncommon situation, when the early onset of psychotic or mood disorder process presents as a developmental delay, misdirecting much needed interventions.

One of the first signs of psychiatric problem could be sleep disturbance: children cannot fall asleep and/or stay asleep, asking adults to stay with them, or coming to their parent's bed in the middle of the night and refusing to sleep alone. As soon as their symptoms subside, they feel comfortable sleeping alone again. Another common sign is the functional impairment at school, behavioral, academic or both. Bright, intelligent children lose the quality of their academic performance, failing, not doing their homework, refusing to go to school, complaining of severe anxiety and demanding their parents take them home in the middle of the day. One of the common and quite misleading diagnoses is "School Phobia", much liked by some school psychologists and pediatricians for its convenience and simplicity. The words "depression" or "anxiety" cause some of the pediatricians quickly give a prescription for one of the popular anti-anxiety anti-depressants like Zoloft, or Celexa, or Lexapro. One of the extreme cases of such treatment of "school phobia" I evaluated a couple of years ago in one of the school districts. A twelve-year-old girl was discharged from a psychiatric hospital after a severe suicidal attempt with an overdose of over the counter medications. She took quite a few tablets of Tylenol and Ibuprofen, and was admitted to the medical floor with the medical complications. She was discharged on no psychotropic medications, but needed to be evaluated by a psychiatrist before allowed to go back to school. When I asked her what happened, she told me that she was getting depressed because of the voices talking to her inside her head, calling her names, putting her down. Her pediatrician gave her Zoloft since her mother reported the signs of depression and ongoing sadness, but never asked her about the reason for her change of the mood. Since this girl started taking Zoloft voices became louder and commanding, telling her she should not live and has to die – which she attempted to do.

Mrs. Mertz: I understand that, but how do you come up with a medical diagnosis and how can we make sense out of this very confusing and controversial picture? Why is it not obvious for everybody that we are dealing not with a spoiled brat, or somebody lost in the fantasy world, but with a sick child?

Dr. A: Psychiatric diagnosis is difficult, especially in children and adolescents. Psychiatry is the only specialty, where the skillful interview remains the main diagnostic tool, same as it was a hundred plus years ago. Some researchers call it "bottom up" interview, which starts from the family history, covers all developmental steps and gradually arrives to the current status of events, looking carefully into all areas of child's life. The onset and development of a mental illness can be better explained using the model of schizophrenia (SCH), as it is one of the most studied psychiatric disorder both in children and adults. One of the latest hypotheses of SCH is called neurodevelopmental, as it states that the abnormality starts from prenatal or perinatal insult, long preceding the onset of clinical manifestation of it. It also includes the role of genetic predisposition and environmental offence. There are numerous studies showing the micro and macro abnormalities in the brain, from discovering genes implicated in SCH, abnormal cell growth, changes in brain neurotransmitters, as well as visible anatomical changes of the brain, indicating the link between maldevelopment and SCH. The incidence of SCH grows from 2-6% in second degree relatives, to 6-17% in first degree relatives, and 50% in identical twins. Only 50%, not all of twins develop SCH, and some patients with SCH do not have any relatives afflicted with this disease. It suggests that environment, not only genetics, could play an important role. Environmental issues include maternal medical conditions, viral infections, Vitamin D deficiency (a very recent study), and labor and delivery complications to mention just a few. The statistics of child's onset schizophrenia is not quite clear; by some reports the onset of schizophrenia before 13 is about 1/30,000. With the "Bipolar Disorder" the situation is far from being remotely clear. Even if a child presents with a pattern of unstable moods, it does not always signify the onset of BD. When I work with adults, I always ask them about their childhood, and the beginning of their emotional problems, as they remember them. All three major categories of adults with either BD, or SCH or schizoaffective disorder almost invariably report the onset of emotional instability, depression, anxiety, mood swings or even ADHD or ODD since their early childhood.

Almost no disease starts abruptly; even an acute infection has several hours of what's called a prodrome, before all symptoms develop at their peak. This prodromal period is a part of any known illness, lasting from several hours to several years. In essence, it presents with nonspecific, vague symptoms of discomfort, tiredness, aches and pains, fatigue etc., when it comes to a physical illness. We all know that many forms of cancer do not manifest themselves until it is too late, as patients tend to ignore their feeling of tiredness or discomfort or explain it with life circumstances. Psychiatric illness is no different, but the prodromal stage would manifest with emotional and cognitive symptoms, or personality changes, which are difficult to link with the coming onset of a psychiatric problem. The "psychiatric" prodrome may start with changes of vitality, decreased level of interest, restrictions of social involvement, academic decline, or out of character behaviors, sometimes with unusual violation of ethics, offensive and impulsive acting out, and many others. If those changes happen around puberty, the most typical response of pediatricians or relatives would be suggestive of developmental issues, need for more discipline, guidance and structure as a universal antidote. It is unlikely that anybody would think about even a remote possibility of a coming mental illness. In medicine we are all for the prophylaxis, but when it comes to psychiatry we try to delay the intervention as much as possible. Could anybody imagine a dermatologist finding a few melanoma cells in skin biopsy and suggesting to wait until it becomes a full blown melanoma? Unlikely; the patient with even one malignant cell will undergo extensive surgery with the radiation or chemo as a follow up. In psychiatry this proper medical approach is reversed: we prefer to sit back and wait until the psychiatric condition becomes so obvious, that nobody has any more doubts about its diagnostic essence. Unfortunately it is much more difficult to treat a full blown psychiatric illness, as the notion of prophylaxis is equally applied to all medical conditions regardless of the "place of their origin".

One of the most confusing prodromal presentations comes in the form of cognitive disorder, which could manifest with processing and attention span problems, working memory deficit, other aspects of intellectual functioning, with a possible drop of IQ over the years (which usually does not draw much attention). Some of those children come with volumes of neuropsychological, psychological, occupational therapy, visual and hearing evaluations, offering different takes and explanation of the problem. Children get diagnoses of Non Verbal Learning Disability, visual and hearing processing problems, motor and coordination problems - to mention just a few. All of those diagnoses are right – because they truly describe what's wrong with a small part of the picture, and wrong – because they do not connect the dots. Neither they give an explanation of the core malfunctioning of the brain, ignoring the fact, that all of the brain functions are intertwined and interlinked, and should not be considered out of the context of the whole picture. Here comes again the Occam's razor phenomenon, stating that out of several competing theories the simplest one truly is the correct explanation. Pages of reports, hours of tests using the cutting edge technology and giving very scientifically sounded diagnoses, carry much more weight, than a psychiatric interview conducted with a pen and paper, and saying that we are dealing with what's called formal thought disorder as a part of a mental illness condition. Simple, but true! Formal thought disorder is a term coming from the classical psychiatry and initially described as an inherent part of schizophrenia. It refers to the inability of the brain to present with logical, sequential and clearly understood way of communication, as well as failure to process and appropriately analyze incoming information. In order to function successfully brain needs to possess different abilities, like processing efficiency, speed of processing, executive function, working memory, self awareness and self regulation. When integrated, those domains constitute the brainpower as well as regulate the functioning and development of different domains of intelligence. Everybody has different ratio of strength and weaknesses; therefore different children and adults have different aptitudes, being more talented in math, or sports, or art. Still all basic abilities of the brain normally are functioning at a proper level, creating the prerequisite of "normal" intelligence. With an early onset of a mental illness different domains of intelligence may suffer earlier, than true psychiatric symptoms become evident. Malfunctioning of different domains would transpire on psychological or other evaluations, but the reason for them, as well as the connection between them will not be detected, until it is deciphered and correlated in the process of a psychiatric evaluation. When the underlying disease is treated appropriately, quite of few of intellectual domains could improve. Sometimes patients who are more attuned to their intellectual performance say that they get "smarter" after their symptoms subside. Recent research showed that patients with schizophrenia show deficits in early auditory and visual processing, contributing to cognitive dysfunction and psychosocial impairment. Specifically it affects the ability to distinguish emotions based on vocal intonation and facial expression. Also reading ability could be severely disturbed. Sensory processing deficits might become a focus of special education arrangement rendering little or no success, because the root of the problem was not detected.

Paradoxically extensive testing might become a barrier, not allowing the child to get appropriate help. Once upon a time I was referred a pleasant adolescent boy, Fred, who came with his mother and a thick file of all possible evaluations performed over the last 8 years, since he was six. He had several psychological and neuropsychological evaluations, occupational therapy and physical therapy treatments, hearing and vision evaluations, multiple special education placements. When we met, he was attending a learning academy, where he was educated on mostly individual basis with a limited exposure to a group of two or three of his peers at a time. His diagnosis given to him by psychologists and his teachers was ADHD, but two medication trials with a stimulant and non-stimulant made him feel worse instead of helping. Unfortunately, even in a highly structured and nurturing environment of his school he was not performing well, getting off task, easily frustrated, angry, banging his fists on the desk, at times talking back and becoming rude. Outside those episodes of frustration triggered by academic difficulties he was quite pleasant and mostly easy going with his family. Another area of concern encompassed his social life: he did not have any friends and did not know how to communicate with his peers, or read social cues, feeling quite alienated and lonely. All of his psychological evaluations unanimously gave him borderline intellectual functioning. When we talked, this young man showed normal intelligence, was able to discuss with me a broad range of topics, demonstrating good reasoning, fund of knowledge, conceptual thinking and keen interest in many areas. We were able to talk about his concentration difficulties not fitting into any diagnostic criteria of ADHD. He had processing troubles consistent with a mild level of thought disorder, as well as lack of impulse control, frustration tolerance, along with some mood shifts. The concentration difficulties stood out, overshadowing other parts of his condition and making everybody think that his lack of focusing was the source of inappropriate behavior. The opposite was true: mood, behavior and processing difficulties (not just the concentration, which is only a part of the thought process) stemmed from the same root of proverbial "chemical imbalance". It was not severe though. Because of the combination of the mild level of mood disorder, fairly high intelligence misrepresented with the "false negative" psychological exam data, and strong school support Fred was able to maintain his level of academic performance.

Mrs. Lawson: What did you recommend and how did he respond to treatment?

Dr. A: I recommended the lowest dose of Risperidone, which could have helped with many facets of his presentation. Needless to say, I explained the dilemma of the lack of black and white indication, diagnostic difficulties for that type of mild disorder, potential ramification of not treating it, especially after the transfer to a regular high school. The parents decided not to proceed with the treatment. They explored on line resources and based on the available data did not feel that Risperidone is the "right" medication for Fred.

Mrs. Lawson: Are you saying that they took upon themselves making a treatment decision not being doctors?

Dr. A: That's exactly what happened; they sent multiple emails after our initial meeting requesting reassurance and more literature sources confirming my diagnostic impression and recommendations. Since I was not able to give them a complete guarantee, that their son is going to be symptom free and well, they decided to stick with behavioral management only. Their position was very difficult: the level of symptoms was not severe from their prospective and the possible side effects and the lack of ironclad information was scary. They opted for what they perceived as a less scary option. The parents did not share my concerns regarding misjudged intelligence and dramatic delay of social skills. They also did not hear my explanations about the limited time we have left, as he was growing older and his brain was getting less resilient, and less able to catch up with missed developmental steps.

Mrs. Mertz: You met with a lot of parents since you became a doctor, probably there are different types of them. I do not share the position of Fred's parents as I do not believe that the medical illness would just disappear without any interventions. What should we do as parents to help our children?

Dr. A: Being a parent is the most difficult and rewarding job! Being a parent of a mentally ill child raises the bar of responsibility and challenges our judgment. Parents become gate keepers of treatment success or failures. Firstly, parents take tremendous responsibility accepting or declining treatment defining their children future. This part applies to all serious medical conditions. I heard from child oncologists about parents angrily leaving their offices, refusing to accept the diagnosis and suggested treatment and therefore jeopardizing their children survival. In psychiatry we mostly talk about the quality of life and safety issues. Untreated mental illness could become deadly because of suicidal or homicidal ideation. Untreated mental illness also can impair the quality of life, development or, if treated early, may cause less or no impact. Either way it is up to the parents to make a decision. The decision is relatively easier when the child is clearly impaired and much more difficult in situations like Fred's. Controlling parents have a more difficult time giving the reigns to somebody else. All parents are given detailed explanations and the rational for the choice of medications as well as an overview of possible side effects. Controlling parents would demand meticulous explanations of every single step, substantiated with multiple literature sources, expecting to be able to compare the data base with their own opinions, which is not possible and not beneficial for their children. They also may not follow the recommendations thinking that "they know their child better." Sometimes the consequences of the latter case scenario could be quite severe. Parents of one of my young patients decided to stop abruptly one of the medications this child took at a low dose. They thought that the medication was not helpful, and stopping this low dose does not pose any risk. As a result the child developed what's called "withdrawal dyskinesia", with repetitive ongoing movements of facial muscles and the tongue. It took a long time and high doses of medications with many more potential side effects to stop those movements. This is a clear example when "playing a doctor" becomes dangerous. It does not happen often though. Fortunately, as difficult as it is, most parents gradually become quite educated in psychiatry and psychopharmacology; they get to understand the connection between doses, types of medications, learn about side effects, and, most importantly, realize that they must not make their own treatment decisions no matter how much they know.

Mrs. Mariebelle: How about this Bipolar Disorder condition? It seems to be the diagnosis of the day! How do we know when it's time to engage a psychiatrist and start the treatment?

Dr. A: That's correct; it appears that the diagnosis of Pediatric

Bipolar Disorder is given frequently and quite liberally. If you see that your child shows emotional problems interfering with the quality of life and developmental success, you should better see a professional and seek a professional opinion. When children develop serious emotional condition, it becomes quite obvious both to the parents and the teachers. You all talked about difficulties finding the right psychiatrist, but it is possible! The situation now is better than it was a decade ago: we have more online support and sources of information along with the names of the psychiatrists. Parents usually exchange information about their "finds" or discourage to repeat their unpleasant experience. You still need to figure out, if the recommended person is right for you and your child. Many factors come into play when you make this decision: does what the doctor says make sense to you, and can he/she communicate clearly all pros and cons of the treatment options, do you feel comfortable asking questions and getting satisfactory answers. A treatment becomes successful if the parents, and the doctor, and, ideally, the child work as a team, discussing victories and failures, exchanging information, observations and thinking together. Children can become very active team players: understaning of the treatment process allows them to "own" the responsibility and grow independence and maturity. Even young children could become amazingly attuned and involved, requesting to increase the dose of the medication, which helped but not enough, or take away another one because it was not useful.

Mrs. Mertz: Are there any scientific data when children should start taking medications and what happens if this optimal time is missed? Will the untreated illness damage the brain forever? Or would the medications damage the brain as well?

Dr. A: It's time to talk about the treatment of psychiatric conditions in children.

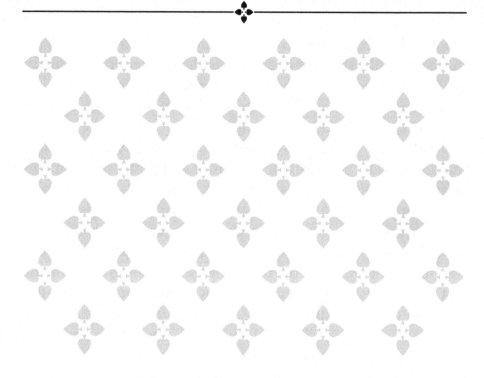

Chapter 8
To Treat or Not to Treat – That Is the Question!

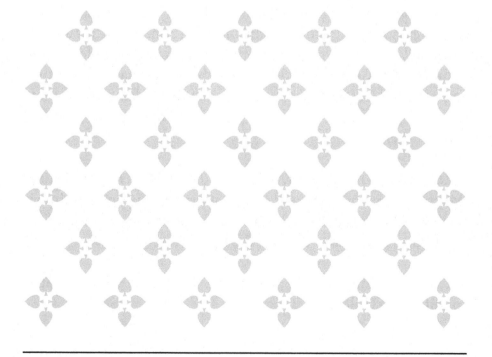

Dr. A: Most of the information about the course and efficacy of treatment is provided by the parents. But the treatment is for children! We seem not to listen enough to them. What do they think about the medications and the personalities of their providers?

My Medicine Journey
By: Jorge Sanchez

Medicine: It all started in April 2005, when I was 9 years old. I was manic and couldn't control myself. I heard voices in my head tolling me to do some crazy things. I listened to them and did what they said. Then, I had to start medicine to control myself. I started Risperdal in April 2005 and that didn't go well. I took 0.5 mg of it and that dose was fine, until I started to take more later on. I started to get calmer, but then I started to gain weight. When I was 7 years old, I was in slim clothes, then after the Risperdal, I needed to wear Husky clothes. After the Risperdal, in May 2005, I started Lexapro, another medicine that actually worked well. I also started off with 20 mg of that. Then I started Lamictal, which I'm still on now. The Lamictal started off at 10 mg. Currently, I'm on 100 mg. The largest dose I've ever taken of it was 125 mg.

In the beginning of 2006, my doctor realized that Risperdal wasn't right for me. I ended it at 2 mg. So then I started Seroquel in the place of Risperdal in mid-2006, which is another medicine I'm still on now. I started taking 100 mg, which is the same dose I'm on now. It worked well, even though I gained a bit more weight.

By November 2007, things became out of control again. I was depressed and couldn't go to school. I started some trial and error medicine, which didn't do anything. Starting in December 2007, I decided I didn't need Lexapro, which actually helped. I didn't know what was good for me back then. I ended it at 30 mg. So, the doctor took me off Lexapro and switched it with Celexa, which started off at 10 mg. I'm currently on the highest dose of 40 mg right now. In December 2007, I tested a medicine called Effexor, which didn't help me at all. I took 37.5 mg of it and I still was the same. In January 2008, I started to feel worse and missed even more school. The doctor kept me out of school for 3 days at the end of January to try some more meds. I tried Abilify, 300 mg of Wellbutrin, 150 mg of Lithium, and 150 mg of Trileptal for a bit of time. None of those worked. I was on those meds for about 2 months. Soon after, I came off of them, which I know I should have done. I also came off of Effexor, which was the longest trial and error med I was on. By June 2008, I missed over 30 days of school, but still passed 6ᵗʰ grade, because I did most of my work at home. By July 2008 I was off all of those trial and error meds and began Invega at 6 mg, which became a long term med that I just came off of in February 2010.

In September 2008, I was on just the Seroquel, Lamictal, Celexa, and Invega. I had trouble starting the 7ᵗʰ grade and didn't make it much after the first day. That was when I began public school and all of the kids were hyper and out of control. I couldn't fit in. After I got a plan in place, I decided I should go after all the kids left for a private tutoring session. I started to get used to the kids and became more comfortable at the school. By November 2008, I was going full day and liking the kids. I also started seeing a helpful therapist, who I still see as of now. By June 2009, when the year ended, I only missed 14 days, a lot less than the previous year.

In January 2010, I had neuropsych testing done. It proved that I didn't have Bipolar disorder or any other things people thought I had. I just was depressed and anxious and I had another kind of problem called Non-Verbal Learning Disorder, which means I have to visualize things instead of verbally hearing about them in order to understand them. It made sense, and I figured out that was the problem and that helped out my grades.

In February 2010, I got off of Invega, which was the last med that

I started in 2008 to get off of. I actually took the last dose of it on my 14th birthday, which was a present for me. Ever since then, I've been fine.

As of September 2010, I'm at a new school, which is high school, and I'm not nervous at all. Currently I'm only on 100 mg of Seroquel, 100 mg of Lamictal, and 40 mg of Celexa, which are helping me and I'm trying to work my way off them.

Help: In 2005 I started to see a therapist named Jerry. He was ok at the beginning, and then when my parents went in to talk to him and tell him about what was going on this past week, he would yell at me to never do that again. More importantly I was only 9 years old. After we got rid of him, in 2006, we saw some other woman named Elaine. She was kind of crazy. We would show up for appointments to find she was not there. Her excuse was "the AC broke". One good thing was that she wasn't mean to me like Jerry was. After her, in 2007, we saw a guy named Dr. K. He wasn't the greatest of all guys, but he was not mean. A better way to describe him is "gruff". We only saw him for a year. Now we're seeing this therapist George since 2008, and he is working out great. Not once has he been mean, not once has he blown us off, and he's not gruff at all. He's great and we're sticking with him for now!

That's my life over the past 5 years. Certainly, a lot goes on in little time!

Dr. A: Jorge presented a very accurate account of his medication trials and his response to them. His problems started at nine with a psychotic episode, when he was hearing voices commanding him to do dangerous things, which he obeyed. Luckily he did not do anything to harm himself or others, which is always the biggest concern. His psychotic symptoms were gradually controlled with medications, but he still was not able to attend the school. After several rounds of different- as he described as "trial and error"-

medications he slowly was improving, returning to school and making his way back to the regular classroom. His medications gradually were tapered, and he is off them completely. Jorge is fourteen now, and given his success, he most likely will be medication free for the foreseeable future. His story is an answer to the question all parents would ask me when we start treatment: "Does it mean that my child is going to be on medications for the rest of the life?" There is no categorical yes or no answer to this question, but quite a few children "outgrow" their symptoms with the help of medications, and can proceed into their adulthood symptom medication free. Most of the parents believe that children require much lower doses than adults, but the situation is exactly the opposite! Children have more liver tissue proportionally to the size of their bodies and more robust metabolism which might require higher doses and more frequent dosing. The closer children approach the adolescence, the more their response to medications becomes similar to that of adults. That is why it is not uncommon to use higher doses in younger kids and lower them in adolescence, as the same dose suddenly is not well tolerated.

Mrs. Anderson: One of my biggest frustrations was that medications were never discussed, as to what we were to watch for in side effects, AND that the medication dose may need to be increased once the child's body got used to the dose. And also for that matter that several medications may be needed to get to the right "cocktail". My younger son was doing very well, then all of a sudden his behaviors were back again with no warning and I was very confused and upset. I did not know that he needed a higher dose, and our psychiatrist would neither see us for another three weeks, nor answer questions over the phone. We were in a crisis mode! Had I known that the meds may have to be increased because of metabolism changes, I would have not felt as helpless.

Dr. A: Yes, in children the clinical picture could change quickly, and that's why we follow them closely, changing the medications and doses to keep symptoms at bay. We need to do it fast, because a lot is happening with the brain tissue in patients with psychotic disorder. The data is more conclusive in adults – the longer is the "life" of psychosis, the more brain volume is lost. Similar data exist for adolescents: they also lose the brain volume as a result of psychotic disorder. Generally, the shorter and "lighter" is the psychotic process, the less is the brain loss. There is no similar data for children for several different reasons. The diagnosis of mental illness in children is not as frequent as in adults. Typically only children with severe psychosis most commonly consistent with the early onset of schizophrenia, or severe mood swings get on the psychiatric radar. Children "hidden" psychoses are commonly misdiagnosed as ADHD, or oppositional defiant disorder, or anxiety, delaying the timely medical intervention. Even when children try to report that something is wrong with them, the adults do not always hear that…

Medication Helps
By K. B.

When I was a child, I had these friends. But no one else could see them. I thought that they were real. To me, they were realer than the family and friends that I had. I honestly thought that they existed. They seemed so realistic.

I loved my friends. But I had enemies too. There was this King Cursor who was trying to kill me because his daughter, Sarah, had left his side to be my friend and protector. He appeared in my room a few times, but my friends would protect me while I cried. I was helpless. I guess these hallucinations really reflected how I felt. I felt afraid that I would always be alone, since the friends that were real were really distant. I was close to my family, but I felt like I was different and that I didn't belong anywhere. I felt that I was useless, unhelpful, unwanted, and unloved. But with my friends, those feelings weren't as bad.

One day, I was talking to my best friend, Sarah. And one of my family members walked in and asked, "Who are you talking to?"

I told them I was talking to Sarah, my best friend, and asked why they had asked that. It was then, for the first time, someone found out about my hallucinations and told me that no one was there. I started yelling for them to stop teasing me, that I could see her that she was there, sitting on my bed.

After that, my friends told me that they weren't alive, that they were spirits, and I was one of the few special people that could see them. It made me feel special. It never really crossed my mind that they weren't real, and that's why no one else could see them. I was reluctant to go on medications. In fact, I despised the idea. I was told it would make my friends go away. And I didn't want that. So, if no one was looking, I didn't take it. I would throw it out or hide it somewhere. But then I was caught hiding them, and had to be watched when I was given my medication. Then I was put on another medication. But this one was for depression.

Then I started getting paranoid. I started thinking that people were going to kill me, or that someone was watching me. And on top of that, I had anxiety issues. It was getting out of control. So I was put on more meds. By this time, my friends the "spirits" were gone. I was sad about that, but I started making connections with real people, so it was for the better.

When I was nine, I tried to commit suicide. I lay down in front of my mother's car, and told her to run me over. I was sent to the emergency room for an evaluation. I was deemed unstable and a danger to myself and was sent to a psychiatric hospital. I was there for a week, and came out feeling a lot better. Some people believe that psychiatric hospitals are for psychopaths and lunatics. But it's meant for anyone with a psych disorder. I have been hospitalized three times, and each time I came out feeling better.

I'm now taking medications for a bunch of different psych issues. And they do help. But right now, my body is going through changes and the meds don't work as well. But as the body changes, often does the way the medications work.

I have been on medications since childhood, and they have helped me tremendously throughout the years. People don't always stay on their medication for their entire lives. People can learn to cope without them. But you first need to try them before you knock them.

Medications really helped me. Without them, I may not be here. I may have killed myself by now because of how unstable I was. I'm truly glad that I started my medication. I started to feel that I was useful, I was helpful, I was wanted, but most of all, I was loved. What else could I ask for?

Mrs. Strom: These are truly amazing stories! Both kids, adolescents now, are so much aware of their problems and have the wisdom to accept the diagnosis and treatment, although it is really hard! And the medications have side effects they are willing to put up with. Do all children go through the same stages? And how do you know what medication is "correct" for the specific patient?

Dr. A: Agreed. Both stories are unique and amazing. The common denominator is the transition from their lives in the world created by their disease to gaining the complete awareness of what is real from what's not. This process is called "insight", and it is usually the best indicator of a good prognosis for the future. The more we are aware of the emotional problems and their roots, the more we invest into recovery with better success. As for the choice of the "right medication" for the patient, let's first go back to the history of psychopharmacology.

Herbal remedies were known to relieve emotional pain since ancient times. One of them was mentioned in the Homer's Odyssey, supposedly opium, which Elena, Zeus daughter, added to the festive drinks, so the guests would forget about their sorrows. In Ellada (Greece) it was believed that the goddess Cerera gave a gift of opium to people in order to free them from sorrow and sufferings. Hashish was used in VIII B.C. by Assyrians. In Peru leaves of cocaine were believed to be sent by gods in order to create the feeling of satiety when hungry, strength when weak, and oblivion of sorrows. Other herbs like Black Nightshade, Henbane, and Atropa as well as alcohol were used as sedatives and sleeping aids. In X B.C. in India Rauwolfia extracted from Rauwolfia Serpentina was used as a sedative and anti-hypertension remedy. Since 1931, it was used for treatment of psychosis, first in India and later in America. In France in the XVIII century Valerian root and Laudanum were used for treatment of mental illness. Coffee and nicotine were considered good for the spirit and mood.

The foundation of contemporary psychopharmacology was laid in 1952 in France. A French surgeon Laborit used Chlorpromazine for treatment of post operative problems and made a serendipitous discovery of its sedative properties. It was used successfully for treatment of manic agitation and other forms of psychosis. Another unexpected discovery was made in patients treated for tuberculosis by Iproniazid, which showed anti-depressive qualities.

Since then the field of psychopharmacology has gotten an avalanche of medications recommended for treatment of different psychiatric conditions. Currently the psychiatric armamentarium consists of multiple medications grouped by FDA approval for psychosis (antipsychotics), depression (antidepressants), mood stabilizers (lithium and anticonvulsants), ADHD medications (stimulants and non stimulants), sedatives, and sleeping aids.

Since the discovery of Chlorpromazine many different chemical groups were investigated and approved for treatment of psychoses. Eventually they were divided into the first generation (FGA), or typical, and the second generation (SGA), or atypical antipsychotics. What is the difference? The typical antipsychotics got their name because they typically induce neurological side effects. They cause the blockade of so called dopamine receptors in the brain, which produce too much dopamine in acute psychotic states. The excessive release of dopamine in the brain was historically connected with the development of schizophrenia and manic phases of bipolar disorder. In order to alleviate psychotic symptoms or mania the level of dopamine should be decreased. But, if the dopamine level gets depleted too much, neurological symptoms similar to Parkinson disease might arise. The atypical antipsychotics do not cause the same level of neurological side effects and target, beside dopamine, a wider range of receptors in the brain putatively involved into development both of schizophrenia and bipolar disorder.

Mrs. Strom: Does it mean that both classes of medications would treat schizophrenia and bipolar disorder? If so, how come they are called antipsychotics, are indicated for the treatment of schizophrenia, but are used for different conditions?

Dr. A: It brings us to the discussion about "on label" vs. "off label" treatment. This is what made Fred's parents so puzzled and distraught. According to the recent studies, only 12 % of psychiatric diagnoses listed in official diagnostic classification have "an approved" drug for their treatment. The rest of them do not have any formally approved or recommended medications. It leaves us with the situation I call "swim at your own risk – no lifeguard on duty". It is even more complicated in child psychiatry: medications approved for adults for the most part are not approved for children. It would take years for FDA to put a stamp of approval on the medications we need to use in child psychiatry. There are many complications in the process of approval, starting with the lack of appropriate classification for child mental illness, difficulties in recruiting patients for treatment arms and control placebo groups, etc. We have to face a dilemma: either to treat the child despite the lack of formal indications, or do nothing, just watching the child decompensating and suffering from long term consequences of untreated mental illness.

Mrs. Mariebelle: How do psychiatrists come to the idea of the off label use of medications? Are you just guessing?

Dr. A: No, there is no guessing involved. We learned over the years, that different psychiatric conditions would cause functional disruptions of the same neurons, creating the notorious "chemical imbalance" in true sense of the word. Imagine a keyboard: by touching different keys you can play different music – jazz, or classic, or spiritual music etc. The keyboard is the same, but the combination of different keys would create different tunes. The brain consists of different neurons and chemicals involved both in normal and disease process. This is the brain "keyboard": different combinations of malfunctioning neurons would be responsible for different psychiatric conditions. For example, the excessive or insufficient amount of dopamine we discussed before is involved in development of schizophrenia, bipolar disorder, depression and ADHD, but its dysregulation happens in different parts of the brain causing different symptoms. When a new medication is released to the market, it has the indication for use along with a detailed description of specific receptors it would affect, or what's called receptor binding profile. You probably saw the commercial for Abilify, describing its indication for treatment of depression. Initially Abilify was approved for treatment of schizophrenia, later it got another approval for bipolar disorder, and then one more approval for depression. When it was used for the treatment of depression with indications for schizophrenia only, it was the "off label" use, now, after the FDA approval for depression, it is "on label". The majority of SGA go through the same sequence of approvals: they got indications for schizophrenia, then for bipolar, and eventually for depression, it is just a matter of time. The knowledge of the receptor predilection as well as the mechanism of action also allows foreseeing possible side effects.

Mrs. Hamilton: How do you choose medications for children, if they do not have the official approval? I would not like to wait until FDA allows using the adult medications for children, but on the other hand, I am concerned about side effects. How do you know, if the medication is safe for children?

Dr. A: Using psychotropic medications for children is one of the most exigent problems. I will not describe in details all medications available on the market, the information is abundant and easily available from multiple different sources, but will try to present a general outline. We do not often use FGA's due to the high incidence of neurological side effects. Mostly we are using SGA's; some of them are approved for children or adolescents, like Risperidone, Abilify, Geodon, Seroquel and Zyprexa. Even before the official approval they were used for treatment of schizophrenia, bipolar or mood disorder "off label" in children and adolescents. When new medications are released to the market, at first we use them as indicated by FDA for specific adult population. Every new medication has a unique profile of receptor affinity, length of life in the body, side effects and other parameters. It takes time for the medication to become integrated into our practices. After psychiatrists gain enough experience with the medication, it ceases being "new" and becomes quite familiar. Now it is possible to introduce it to child and adolescent psychiatry. Many variables are taken into consideration when we choose medications for children. There are two facets of safety: one is the safety of the medication in terms of its short and long term side effects, and another is the "safety" of leaving the undertreated or resistant to treatment condition. When "old" medications work we do not change them. The need for change comes only when the symptoms of severe mental illness do not subside affecting the quality of life. Mrs. Mariebelle: How safe are psychotropic medications?

Dr. A: "Safe medication" is an oxymoron. No medication is safe, including OTC and herbal supplements or remedies. Parents would never look into the side effect list of favorite OTC medications and liberally give their children Tylenol, cough medicines and such. They would be appalled to discover, that all of them have severe side effects, including gastric bleeding, kidney and liver failures, psychosis, dependence and addiction etc. Parents of one of the children currently in treatment with me were extremely apprehensive about psychotropic medications and inconsistent about their decisions, which eventually caused the increase of the baseline symptoms and development of paradoxically more side effects. But they did not hesitate to put the child on a high dose of Benadryl, because it is available without a prescription. Benadryl caused its own side effects and created a physical dependence, so each time when we attempted to lower the dose side effects got worse. Taking the child off Benadryl became a separate challenge, besides treating the preexisting mental illness. The parents were understandably upset, admitting that they never looked into the spectrum of side effects, just assuming, that if Benadryl is OTC it is safe to use. Somehow when we talk about a prescription medication everybody is eager to look it up on line and form an opinion (mostly negative), but it does not apply to non-prescription remedies. The same is true about SAM-e, which has some severe side effects and especially drug-drug interaction, Ginseng, Valerian root – the list could be continued indefinitely. We live in an era of educated consumers, which is a mixed blessing. Of course, information and knowledge are power, but when it is misplaced it becomes a barrier to successful treatment outcome. Children and adolescents are even more skillful then their parents, finding on line all information about medications they take or supposed to take. My eleven-year-old patient was misdiagnosed with ADHD and unsuccessfully treated with stimulants, making his condition much worse. I suggested starting him on a very low dose of Risperidone, indicated for a variety of different reasons. He looked it up and refused to take it because on line he read it was recommended for schizophrenia and might cause tardive dyskinesia. He did not have schizophrenia, but had Autistic spectrum disorder with a high level of aggression, which is one of the indications for Risperidone. Still he refused, and his parents were not able to convince him. This is an example of how the knowledge becomes "pseudo knowledge". There is an old joke. One lady asked a doctor: "Why do your patients need to see you, if we can read a medical book and figure out the treatment ourselves?" To which the doctor responded: "Because there is a chance to die because of the typo." This is very true, because in order to become a doctor we need to go through many years of different types of formal training, which does not ever end until we retire. The diagnosis and treatment recommendations are based on many "layers" of knowledge and experience that cannot be just acquired from reading a book or even many books. Nobody expects to become a gourmet chief after reading and cooking a recipe from a cook book, or becoming an expert in mechanics after reading about fixing a car on line. You probably agree that the health is more complicated and eventually may be irrevocably damaged if mishandled. There is a thin line when too much education gives our patients the false impression, that they know as much as the doctors and can disregard any medical advice, or change their treatments without consulting their medical professionals.

Mrs. Anderson: I understand this, but still it is scary to trust the life and well being of our children into hands of somebody we do not know! How do we know the doctor is making the right decision if we are not well informed? How do we know that we need to use medications and how can we find the "right doctor"?

Dr. A: Both are crucial questions with no black and white answers. Starting a child on any medication is always a hard decision. Not all conditions should be medicated: we learned how to hastily use "big guns", introducing Prednisone at the first sign of asthma, and antibiotics for a common cold, or ADHD medications when a child is not doing well at school, neglecting to appraise all potential side effects. We need to treat a medical condition, if it is a threat to life and well being, or if it significantly impedes the quality of life, slowing the child development. The use of Prednisone is crucial in severe asthma, and antibiotics are necessary for strep throats, but if used for mild symptoms both might cause more side effects than benefits. The definition of necessary vs. optional in child psychiatry is even more complicated and based on the agreement between a trusted provider, parents, and preferably the child as well. Let's start with ADHD as a model of a psychiatric condition. There are shades of grey: some children have signs of it, but can perform well at school with some additional accommodations like seating preference, extended time for quizzes and tests in a quiet room, at times extra tutoring. They also do not suffer developmentally; have appropriate social life and chose extracurricular activities in structured and dynamic settings. Obviously medications are optional for those types. On the other hand, there are children or adolescents who cannot maintain their attention or focus for a split second despite their high intelligence. They "lose" it at school and socially, not learning academically and missing developmental social cues falling behind their peers. For those youngsters medications are more mandatory, as the untreated child would miss important development steps without a chance to catch up in the future, at times having high but "inaccessible" IQ. These are two extremes on the spectrum of events with multiple transitional conditions in between. The key question, which should help you choosing the right direction, is: to what extent the medical condition interferes with the normal life and development of the child? When our children have high fever, it does not take long to make a decision to keep them home and take them to a pediatrician, because we know that the child would not be able to perform at school. You can always use this analogy comparing the emotional/mental condition of your child with "fever" and take steps when it is really "high".

The psychotropic medications have serious side effects. Some of them are what's called "class side effects", as neurological side effects of all antipsychotic medications, more frequent with FGA and less so with SGA. Quite a few medications are causing weight gain and sedation regardless of their class. Also some medications have "signature" side effects, making them different from others in their class. For example, Risperidone, approved for some childhood psychiatric conditions, causes elevation of hormone prolactin. This is a well known and well studied side effect, which can be safely managed. Because we know that it may happen we watch closely for any early signs of it and switch to a different drug if needed. Other side effects may not be that easy to get rid of, but usually when we take care of them early enough, they would not persist. Also when we start a child on a new medication we recommend the lowest possible dose and increase it gradually, watching for possible side effects or intolerance.

Mrs. Lawson: What do we do with the weight gain? I noticed that my children tend to eat more since they were put on medications, subsequently gaining more weight. There is also a diabetes warning for almost all medications. Does it mean that everybody taking Risperidone or Zyprexa or other drugs would develop diabetes?

Dr. A: Many medications cause weight gain by increasing appetite and slowing metabolism. We do not know exactly why it happens, although there are several hypotheses. Still we cannot address this problem out of context of the general trend in the population. According to CDC (Center for Disease Control), the incidence of obesity and diabetes in US is on the rise. In some states the rate of child obesity approaches almost 30%. High weight becomes a risk factor for diabetes. CDC offers several explanations for this phenomenon. Children tend to spend more time in front of TV and computers, leading sedentary life style, eat sugary snacks and junk food, not controlling their portions. Schools have vending machine selling sugary beverages and snacks. So, it comes to the combination of high caloric intake along with insufficient burning of consumed calories. If we eat more than we burn, the extra calories turn into fat; if we eat and burn in equal measure we maintain our weight, and if we eat less than burn we lose weight. This is a simple equation helping to understand the mechanics of gaining and losing weight. Children and adolescents spending more time outdoors or involved into sports tend to eat healthier and burn more energy not gaining weight or even losing it.

Mrs. Anderson: Do you recommend any diets?

Dr. A: Not really. Losing weight on a diet and then gaining it back, when the "diet mood" is over, is not helping. The concept of "a diet" does not sit well with many of us, as it means restrictions and deprivations, or too much work in the kitchen and thinking about what and when to eat. Portion control along with several small meals a day, with the emphasis on fruit, vegetable, protein and whole grains work as well as any diet. It is not a diet per se, but rather a different life style, which eventually helps the body to learn different eating habits, decrease the weight and sustain it. Needless to say that physical activity and sufficient hydration are inherent parts of the plan.

Mrs. Mertz: How could we manage our children and especially adolescents if they refuse taking medications? What do you say to an adolescent who is not willing to take anything and does not believe that medications might help?

Dr. A: Children seem to be easier to convince: they may have specific concerns or dislikes of the taste or the size of the pill. In those cases "a tablespoon of sugar makes the medicine go down": a tablespoon of ice cream or apple sauce would make wonders to the compliance with the treatment plan. Some children cannot take pills, and we can prescribe either liquid forms or crush some of the tablets. With adolescents everything is more testing: sometimes the disease is gone too far, they lose the insight and have to be admitted to the hospital and started on medication there. When their condition improves, they get to understand their illness, making a connection between taking medications and feeling better, and usually become more cooperative. Sometimes they have a negative experience with medication and lose any faith in treatment. In those cases it is truly difficult, as they cannot be admitted if not symptomatic enough, and are quite hostile toward their parents and psychiatrists. One of my patients, a young adult now, came to my practice when she was an angry and rebellious adolescent, terrorizing the household, physically assaulting her parents and getting arrested for that. Before we met, she was treated for "ADHD", which she had to some extent, but was not treated for severe mood swings, anger, and depression. The parents complained that she has never been compliant with her medications, always sabotaging any treatment approaches. The girl failed high school, attending a special education programs for many years, and, to dismay of her parents, did not show any interests or plans to have a meaningful life in the future. She was quite tense and hostile to me as well: it took time to develop a relationship with her. She became an ally and the team player after I redirected all treatment responsibilities to her: she was in charge of taking medications, ordering refills and providing me with the feedback about her progress. She has never been treated this way: usually her parents offered a long list of complain to her psychiatrists, and she was just present there. In my office she discovered, that even with her parents present at our meetings, she is the one making most of the decisions. It took us some ups and downs, but she graduated from high school, successfully took several college courses, and worked a couple of jobs at a time, eventually launching out into a highly competitive career. She is in control of her symptoms now, not willing to change any of her meds. The turning point for her was the realization, that she had a complicated medical condition, and that I was offering my help to her, not her parents. Most of the adolescents want to be heard and helped, but it takes time and effort to establish a connection and get their trust.

Mrs. Mariebelle: Is there any data about video games, especially violent, and their influence on children's behavior?

Dr. A: So far no connection has been established between violent videogames and aggressive behavior. On the other hand, depression was linked with aggression and antisocial behavior in youth. Video games though could become addictive: both children and adolescents, especially those with emotional problems, end up encapsulating themselves in a bubble of ongoing interaction with a computer or videogame system. It is not unusual to hear about battles over the video/computer games, when children become consumed with playing to the exclusion of any social interaction or homework. This preoccupation with videogames can become another symptom of disease, as well as any other self admi-nistered, sometimes street, "remedy" alleviating the emotional discomfort. In any case it must be brought up and discussed with the psychiatrist.

Intermission

Dr. A: Let me ask our panelists: what would you advise to the parents suspecting or having children with mental illness? As we all agreed, hearing this diagnosis is an overpowering experience to begin with. The resourses are limited, as our society is not ready and willing to accept mental illness as a medical condition and treat it as such. There is still a stigma attached to any mental problem, which is viewed as disgrace, or family flaws, which is not true in the first place, and interferes with getting appropriate help fast. If you can imagine yourself in the shoes of "psychiatrically naïve" parents, how would you redirect them for help?

Mrs. Strom: As I ponder the question of what we would advise parents who are beginning a similar journey, my mind wanders to a friend I knew in high school. I recently saw her in a store, and she shared her son's diagnosis of autism in the form of Asperger's syndrome. The diagnosis was only several days old, and her pain was still raw. The grief, shock and fear were still overpowering everything else. If you are in that spot and the diagnosis is fresh, take some time to grieve and give yourself a break. This stuff is scary, possibly one of the scariest things you may ever have to face. Your child has an illness that is potentially debilitating and progressive. The long term future may seem uncertain. Allow yourself to grieve; you are no less of a person for it, and a child with mental illness does not make you a failure as a parent. You were no more able to control this than controlling what color your children's eyes are. What you can control though is making sure, that your child gets help. Praise yourself for recognizing a problem, since knowing is the beginning of working towards a goal and treatment. In our experience, we have seen several parents who have denied that a problem could possibly exist within their child. They blamed everyone, from teachers to caregivers from the earliest years. Ultimately though, blaming others did nothing to help their child If anything, we have learned that it is better to intervene at the earliest point voluntarily, rather than wait until you are forced to by the school or social community. Yet even if you have waited, it's still never too late. My husband's favorite saying is: "Just do something, even if it's wrong!" I truly believe that parents have an innate ability to know a problem exists long before anyone else sees it. It is important to always follow the intuition of your inner voice and your heart.

So, our first suggestion is just what we wrote above; seek help. Speaking of help, we would say: see your pediatrician first. From there you may progress to a therapist, psychiatrist, psychologists, etc.; whomever you may need to see, based on the professionals' recommendations. Your child needs you to take that step towards help for them. Only you are your child's best helper and advocate. Teachers and such are advocates, but almost no one can replace you getting help for your child.

Our second suggestion is to find support. By support, we mean anyone you can trust with your fears, progress and setbacks. This may be a family member, neighbor, internet, community, or faith based support group, or another parent. It doesn't need to be a large group; it can be only one or two other people. I received more support and knowledge from one woman, than I may have received from twenty, who had never experienced my particular pain and suffering of having a child with mental illness. At some point you are going to need this type of assistance to help you with everything, from emotional support, to medical questions, and navigating educational laws. You may find a group, where support is given to parents of children suffering from any medical condition, but - if possible- try to find someone or a group of people, who have children suffering from similar mental illness. Many times just finding others, who are on the road you are on, will give you the hope and strength you need at the moment you need it.

Thirdly, get a game plan if your child's illness causes undesirable behaviors, and do yourself a favor by forgiving people now. Eventually you will find yourself in a situation, where a person is judgmental or critical, whether it is a family member, teacher, or complete stranger. Prepare yourself for those situations ahead of time: it allows you to become a better educator and advocate for your child. I know a parent, who chooses to educate by hand-ing out a small card with information explaining their sons disorder, and asking for compassion, if he becomes agitated in a social setting. Ralph Waldo Emerson said: "For every minute you are angry you lose sixty seconds of happiness." Prepare your strategy and make up your mind now, that you will not let this illness, diagnosis, or opinions of other people rob you of your happiness.

And finally, if we can offer anything, it would be to remember to take one day at a time and not to lose hope. For us, our hope has been and remains Christian hope. We put our trust in God's promises and have confidence in Him. Dr. Harold Wolff, professor of medicine at Cornell University Medical College, spoke about not despairing and having hope. He said: "Hope, like faith and a purpose in life is medicinal. This is not a statement of belief, but a conclusion, proved by meticulously controlled scientific experiment." We have found that treating mental illness can sometimes feel like you are chasing the wind. We recommend taking a deep breath, and persevering. Ann Landers, the incomparable advice giver, summed it up nicely when she said: "If I were asked to give what I consider the single most useful bit of advice for all humanity, it would be this: expect trouble as an inevitable part of life and when it comes, hold you head high, look it squarely in eye and say, 'I will be bigger than you. You cannot defeat me.'"

Mrs. Anderson: I agree with all of that: the first thing that comes to mind is finding competent medical resources in all arenas, including pediatric care, psychological and psychiatric care, and appropriate therapeutic programs including Physical Therapy, Speech and Language, and Behavioral therapies. Once these providers are in place, it is important that they communicate with each other (which sometimes is a problem by itself!). Once you have your medical team in place, you can set appropriate level of educational expectations of your child. You must say to yourself, that you are the parent of a special needs child, and you make decisions. While your medical providers as well as the education community are experts in their fields, in the end, it will be you, based on their advice, making the decisions for your child. And it is you, who will be paying for these services, be it in insurance co-pays, out of pocket, or by paying your city and state taxes.

I found myself sitting in so many classrooms and watching education administrators doing their jobs to make sure that they did their jobs right – and I was not getting paid to do this. I learned to not be intimidated by the "experts", and began questioning them on what they intended to do for my child, how they intended to it, what results were to be looked for, and in what time frame should I expect to see the results. And I expected the answers from teachers all the way up to district superintendents, therapists, and lawyers. Take control, document everything, and do not be afraid to hold the "experts" accountable for what they say they are going to do for your child. And do not be afraid of any retribution from the school districts pertaining to your other children in other classes. It is against the law and really, they should be very alert that you are watching them and that you will not hesitate to call them out on the carpet. Be respectful, stand back, and watch. Empower yourself with knowledge, it is a better use of your time than wasting energy being upset about things you could have known about to help your child.

Teasing out behavior is another challenge. When one of the boys is displaying inappropriate behavior, I go through the following litany in my head:

Is this behavior medical, related to current medications?

Is this behavior a result of the disability?

Is the child just being a nasty brat who needs to have a nap or go into a time out?

This litany is so important that you need to use it as your mantra. Before we truly understood the behaviors associated with the boys' disabilities, we could not understand why they kept behaving the way they were. Using what we learned growing up, there were lines drawn in the sand, that a child just did not cross and behaviors that are simply not acceptable. When David or Ben misbehaved, they got punished. It was time out time and strict voice time. Time and time again, instance, after instance, after instance, and we just didn't get it. It wasn't until we began to uncover the diagnoses, until we began to understand the behavior patterns associated with the diagnoses and our child, and then we began to figure out how to deal with the behaviors. We are still working on this however. Ben has a perseveration problem, and he cannot let go of an idea when it is something that he wants. He will continue to ask again, and again, and again in high hopes that the answer will change. This can become really annoying after the tenth time of saying we are not going out to dinner. We want to scream, but alas, that will only exacerbate the situation. The perseveration is the result of his disability, and it is our job to teach him to lessen his anxiety and get over the fact, that we are not going out to dinner.

It is also critical to maintain this mantra when educating the educational community about your child's disability. If behavior issues come up at school, then you must assist them in understanding the root of the behavior. Better you make that call, and then allow them to dole out a punishment out of ignorance that will unlikely fit the crime.

Mrs. Strom: We are "seasoned" parents, but still have questions and I'm not sure that they really have any answers. One thing that my husband and I have discussed is what will the teenage years hold. We have heard horror stories from other parents as they have looked at us, smiled and said "just wait...it gets much worse". How in the world can we prepare or brace ourselves for when our child hits puberty. Will it be as bad as the nightmares we are envisioning? I had one parent sarcastically telling me: "Just wait until his first hospitalization, that's how you will know your hell has begun." Another question along those lines would be: does anyone actually outgrow this? I mean have anybody ever seen anyone, even one patient who was like our child/children who eventually turned out normal?" (By "normal" I mean no diagnosis of adulthood psychiatric illness).

Chapter 9
What Does the Crystal Ball Say?
What Does Science Say?

Dr. A: Both questions are somewhat related to each other. Let me start with the hospital admission "horror". Of course, the whole process of going to the hospital, sometimes via ambulance, spending hours in the ER, is a scary experience for the child and traumatic for the parents. This is an extreme step, which we take only if the child is highly symptomatic, in danger of self harm/harm to others, has intense auditorial hallucinosis, with voices commanding to act in a dangerous way, or agitated and impossible to contain at home. As unpleasant as it is, an inpatient admission could be therapeutic, putting the child in a safe environment and sending a message that scary things nobody else can see or hear, torturing the brain have a medical foundation, and could be treated as any other medical condition. A psychiatric admission is no different from any other medical one: we have such a deep sitting stigma of a psychiatric diagnosis, that everything remotely connected with it is perceived as spooky and disgraceful. Consider a situation when a child has a spike of fever or an asthma attack. As parents we try to calm the child, put him or her in a comfortable environment without any excessive stimuli. Also we give medications recommended by the doctor for those occasions. If we deal with a child who has a "spike" of acute agitation caused by a mood swing, or increase of psychotic symptoms, the usual way to deal with it is… punishment! At the very best, the child will be put in a timeout room getting scornful comments from teachers for "bad" behavior. Unfortunately the child is not more responsible for this behavior than for the fever or asthma attack. I get questions how to handle an agitated child at home and at school time and again from parents and teachers. First and foremost the child shouldn't feel that he or she is misbehaving and is being punished. Moving into a quiet room is a must at school, but the child should be supervised by an adult at all times; it will not be a good idea to leave an agitated child to "cool down" alone. Distraction may work quite well (same principle as comforting a child with high fever); usually teachers know quite well what this child likes. It could be a snack, or a drink, or some favorite activities like coloring or even

10-15 minutes of video games. At home parents can follow the same steps. As Mrs. Anderson described, dealing with any kind of abnormal behavior, even with the knowledge that it is a symptom of illness, is difficult and taxing. Children suffering from a mental illness quite commonly become preoccupied with certain activities, whether it is dining out, or going to a store, or getting a pet. They demand to get what they want relentlessly, disregarding the "no" answer and just getting more agitated. Still parents know their children preferences and can use them as distractions. Switching the attention of the child to something else, less desirable, but still enticing could do the trick. For example, if dining out is out of the question, an extra snack or a brief break for a video game could become a saving grace. Needless to say, that the policy of mutual compromise should not open the door to ongoing manipulative behavior. This is one of the situations that could be productively discussed in the frame of family therapy, or with an individual child therapist, especially when the child is not in the middle of the emotional crisis and has more insight into his or her problematic behaviors.

Most of the emergency room visits with anxious or agitated children entail hours of waiting, after which the episode ends by itself, and the patient is released home with recommendation to see the outpatient psychiatrist for a follow up visit. Less frequently children are being admitted, only if their behavior would pose any ongoing risk for them or others, or if they are grossly symptomatic, showing signs of severe psychosis. To avoid the unpleasantness and frustration of unnecessary trips parent can discuss with their psychiatrists medications to control the agitation. Sometimes it could be an extra dose of the medication the child takes on a regular basis; sometimes it is a different sedative (often the same one prescribed in ER).

The question about "outgrowing" the mental illness is more complicated. Of course, we all would like to have a peek into the future, especially when our children's life and wellbeing is at stake. In the absence of a crystal ball let's try to look into some scientific data.

According to the latest studies, there is a close connection between the process of neuronal pruning happening in adolescence and the onset of mental illness. What does it mean? The child is born with "overproduction" of many structural elements of the brain, including neurons and connections between them. It is called "the overshooting phenomenon", which provides exceptional plasticity, allowing the brain to adapt to different environmental factors and refine itself. Until recently, most scientists believed that the major "wiring" of the brain was completed by as early as three years of age, and that the brain would be fully mature by the age of ten or twelve. Recent research by scientists at the National Institute of Mental Health (NIMH), using magnetic resonance imaging (MRI), has found that a brain is still developing during the teen years and even continues into the 20's. The period of creating connections between brain cells and their pruning extends from just before birth through adolescence. From early youth to prepuberty the number of connections is stable, but undergoes reorganization. Around puberty 30%–40% of synapses are removed. In the best case, this reorganization leads to a stable adult synaptic network. Most surprisingly, the brain gets a second wave of overproduction of gray matter, something that was thought to happen only in the first eighteen months of life. Following the overproduction of gray matter, the brain undergoes a process called "pruning", where connections among neurons in the brain that are not used are snipped away, while those that are used frequently stay — the "use it or lose it" principle. It is thought that this pruning process makes the brain more efficient by strengthening the connections used most often, and eliminating the clutter of those that are not used at all. In one of the studies, repeated MRI scans revealed increased cortical thickness during childhood followed by thinning of the cerebral cortex proceeding from the back to the front during adolescence. As the cortex gets thinner, the underlying myelin content of the white matter increases. It was suggested that effective pruning increases brain efficiency, and superior intelligence correlates with an initial accelerated, prolonged phase of cortical increase in children followed by equally vigorous cortical thinning by early adolescence. The pruning process is dynamic and profound.

What does this mean for teens? According to scientists, it is during these biological changes that teens may actually be able to control their own brains. Children may want to hard-wire their brain for sports, music or math, i.e. strengthening the connections by using them more often, or lose them by lying on the couch in front of the television and playing video games, either way laying the foundation for their future. Synaptic pruning is thought to help the brain transition from childhood, when it is able to learn and make new connections easily, to adulthood, when it is more settled in its structure, can focus on a single problem for longer, and carry out more complex thought processes. We tend to "demonize" adolescents, anticipating the worst possible problems coming with this age, often seeing just the rebellious and nonconforming behavior. The truth is that adolescence is a true separation-in-dividuation stage of life, with many exciting possibilities. This is the time of transformation of an ugly duckling into a beautiful swan, when the vast connectivity of the brain temporarily coexists with the adult oriented tasks, creating the underpinning for successful learning.

On the other hand, the adolescent brain is very sensitive to the harmful effects of alcohol: the research has shown that heavy, on-going alcohol use by adolescents can impair cognitive brain functioning compared with non-abusing peers, even weeks after they stop drinking. This suggests that abuse of alcohol by teens may have long-term negative effects on the structure and development of their brains.

Teens also differ from adults in their ability to read and understand emotions in the faces of others. Recent research shows that teens and adults use different regions of the brain when responding to certain tasks. Synaptic pruning is just one of many changes thought to be going on inside teenager's brains. It was found that teens cannot multitask as well as adults, because their brains are still learning how to process multiple pieces of information at once, the way adults can. In addition to changes that affect how they think, teenager's brains also undergo developments that affect how they feel. For example, during adolescence teens begin to empathize more with others, and take into account how their actions will affect not just themselves, but people around them. On the other hand, frontal cortex, the part of the brain associated with higher level thinking, empathy, and guilt, is underused compared to adults. But as adolescents mature, they begin to use this region more when making decisions, indicating that they increasingly consider others when making choices.

This extensive connectivity and overproduction of neurons plays another very important role. If a child receives a brain injury before age ten, because of the huge brain "network", another area of the brain can often take over the functions of the damaged region. If the same injury occurs at age twenty, however, the person may lose a vital ability, because the brain has lost the flexibility and pathways to transfer that function to another area. This process is the biological substrate and the explanation of why young children can learn a foreign language without an accent, or why they can learn the sports, or music to become professionals only at a certain young age.

In the worst case, this pruning could disable the individual and sometimes lead to mental illness. Errors in pruning happen in some teens, but little is known about the kind of errors that occur. We can only speculate why some teens emerge with better brains and others emerge with brains that do not function well. It has been hypothesized than mental disorders might be connected to the pruning of the neural networks of the developing brain. When the pruning is shut down too soon (early maturers), the synaptic density will be high and could be subject to mutual electrochemical influences. These tend to synchronize the neighboring neurons, which might be locked into a pattern of paroxysmal activity, which complicates the CNS function. In contrast, in late maturers the synaptic density will be below optimal, because of the failure to shut down the pruning process. The reduced synaptic density and the associated tendency to desynchronization could lead to a general breakdown of circuitry. There are hypotheses saying that both too early and too late shut down of the pruning process could lead to mental disorders. In early maturers, manic-depressive psychosis is more common, while late maturers more often get schizophrenia.

This kind of structural changes that normally occurs in the neural networks of the brain throughout life is also apparent at later stages in life, as the adaptability or learning capacity of the brain is gradually weakened. This is, of course, particularly apparent in dementia, such as Alzheimer's disease, where learning is severely impaired. Also strokes and lesions of various sorts can affect a natural and healthy balance between stability and flexibility, between order and disorder in our neural and mental processes. Thus, there should be a balance between stability and flexibility that ensures an efficient information processing.

The frontal lobe of the brain, especially prefrontal cortex (PFC) is involved in what is known as "executive functioning". It allows us to pay attention and use our working memory holding several facts or thoughts in memory temporarily, while solving a problem or performing a task. Synapses are gaps between nerve cells in the brain which allow important connections within the brain. Research is suggesting that synaptic connections within the PFC may be disturbed in schizophrenia. Many of the functions of the PFC take a while to develop – usually until late teenage or early adulthood years – times considered to be of vulnerability and opportunity. It was suggested that in schizophrenia, during these critical teenage/early adulthood years, there may be disruptions in synaptic pruning in the PFC. Such disturbances in normal brain development may then either directly trigger or indirectly contribute to the onset of schizophrenia symptoms. It was also speculated that there may be functional unmasking of preexisting synaptic deficits by an otherwise normal synaptic pruning process.

Apparently, this complex and challenging adolescent behavior has a powerful biological underpinning, explaining at least some of the problems we encounter as parents. Is it really that "horrible" as a friend of Mrs. Strom indicated? I do not think so! It is difficult; it takes a lot of patience and understanding to deal with a, so to speak, normal adolescent. Needless to say, that in an adolescent with any mental disease all problems would be augmented. In the past, practicing psychiatrists noticed that the onset of a psychiatric illness happens usually around puberty – not knowing anything about the neuronal pruning and molecular restructuring of the brain. In my own experience, quite a few of the patients, who started treatment early enough, were able to grow into high functioning young adults without taking any medications, which is consistent with the concept of reprogramming the brain when it still has a vast network of neuronal connections.

Mrs. Strom: Another question that my husband has posed in the past is that if science can show the levels of certain chemicals in the brain are abnormal in mental illness, why can't we just regulate those particular chemicals? It is frustrating to parents that we can put a man on the moon, but can't find a way to determine how to scientifically test and regulate the levels of chemicals in our brains. How far off realistically are we from this kind of diagnostic/treatment option?

Dr. A: The levels of chemicals in the brain and in the peripheral blood are different. The brain has its own independent state of equilibrium, producing and receiving nutrients and chemical from blood, and is protected with so called blood-brain barrier strictly censoring ins and outs. So far we cannot have a blood test, accurately reflecting the neurochemical shift in the brain. There are some theories regarding preventive strategy changing the course of developmental events in those, who are at high risk. It concerns patients in prodromal stages of the illness, which means before the actual onset of psychotic symptoms. Some authors go into details pertaining to the brain chemistry and circuits that might be involved, suggesting medications potentially manipulating the synaptic pruning problem. However, so far there are just theories proposed by the authors, and much more research and testing is needed to see whether different drugs are able to help in preventive efforts. Regardless, we need to have a much better understanding of what is going on at the smallest of levels in the brain – cellular and molecular – in order to generate hypotheses of new preventive and therapeutic strategies that can perhaps help in prevention efforts. Ironically, sending people to the moon is easier, than understanding what's going on inside the brain on the molecular and cellular levels and interfering with those processes.

Mrs. Strom: What do we tell society in general? It seems every time we turn around, there is another article or news story highlighting how childhood mental illness (from ADHD to bipolar disorders) is being over diagnosed. They negate the reality and proof that childhood mental illness and the suffering of these families are real. The inferences are devastating to parents fighting to change how people view their children and mental illness in general. How should we respond to parents and educators, who read a quote in our local newspaper, where the superintendent of schools said that most special needs kids in the district are the offspring of drug addicts and products of neglect, whose parents are abusing the system? Every time someone reads these things, it makes it easier for educators, those with "normal" children, and society in general to pass negative judgments.

Dr. A: Historically mental illness for years remained an invisible, intangible condition, which was supposed to be managed either by sheer will power, or changes in the parental techniques, or family structure. Only now, through pain and frustration, we are gradually coming to the realization that psychiatric problems like other diseases have medical origins. Negative judgment and prejudice come from the lack of knowledge and education. Nobody makes a secret out of asthma; the school nurse usually has instructions and inhalers to use, if a child has an attack. Parents of children with mental illness would agonize about how much they can disclose to the school and their friends. Recently I saw a six-year-old child, presenting with a quite typical picture of severe mood swings, aggressive behavior, making the life of the whole family unhappy. Since he was put on Risperidone, his behavior and mood improved dramatically. For the first time the family had a normal vacation, enjoying their trip instead of crying, screaming, and yelling. Still this child remained academically behind, and was offered a summer school. At the same time, at his PPT the school psychologist, talking about possible learning disability, refused to conduct a psychological evaluation or approve special education services. The frustrated mother asked how far she should go, pushing the psychological evaluation, and how much she needs to disclose to the school, fearing that her child would be stigmatized for the next twelve years. What would you say?

Mrs. Strom: Our situation with son #1 mimicked that of this parent, only the school was aware of his medications. He made little academic progress in Kindergarten in the way of reading. In first grade, they offered "special reading interventions", but by the end of first grade little progress was made. The school was very resistant to having him tested when we requested it. They stated that for the ease of their schedules and annual reviews, they normally do not test until 2nd grade at age seven. We conceded and essentially first grade became a completely wasted year, where he fell significantly more and more behind academically. Teachers privately admitted to us, that this rule of testing often leads to just a period of wasted "waiting" for many children. They know ultimately, that this student needs special education, but because they are bound by the rules and directions of their superiors, they are essentially helpless to the system. We then sent him to a summer reading program between 1st and 2nd grade, which was not only frustrating to him, but led to absolutely no academic gains. At the beginning of second grade we were insistent that he be tested at the very beginning of the school year. The result of the schools testing unfortunately was as equally flawed as the system. We felt, when the results were read, that the teachers looked extremely pressured and uncomfortable reading their findings. In fact, the school psychologist actually broke out in a case of hives all over her neck and face while she was presenting her findings! They said that their findings indicated no need for special education services (contrary to what they all discussed privately with us). We fought them, refuted the findings and requested a formal neuropsychological evaluation from an independent psychologist. The school board conceded to the formal testing, and indeed our son presented with significant learning disabilities, that required very specialized education services. The findings recommended a specialized reading program at that point not offered in our school system. It was because of our pressure, that the Board of Education instituted training special education teachers in this reading program, and it is now offered city wide to many other students who require it.

The first matter I would recommend for this parent is to decide if they wish to disclose the medication the child is on. Two things we realized early were that it is never healthy to be embarrassed that your child is on medications. Not that this is the case for this parent, but I am no more embarrassed that my child is on psychiatric medications, than I would be if my child were an insulin dependent diabetic. He needs it, it helps him, and that is that. Even if it is transient and not lifelong, I never want him to believe, that I am in any way ashamed of him or his illness. No matter what you do or say, there will always be people that have pre-conceived notions and judgments, within the school system, the community and our families. Often times, disclosing privately that your child is on medications to the team solidifies and substantiates, that this child has special education needs. Sometimes, being on medications can help qualify the child for special education under the Other Health Impaired label. Also I always recommend to parents of children with special needs to decide early on what your goals are for this child, and stick to your guns! Do you know in your heart or gut that your child needs more, than main stream education can provide? Do you suspect a learning disability? Do you feel, that simply pulling the child out of the class for "extra help" is not going to be enough? Then decide that you will not be a slave of the system, and fight for the testing, despite the opposition you will receive. You are not doing your child any favors by backing down and believing that that the "educators" know best. If a parent requests the testing, the school needs to do it! Resist the scare tactics they use and do what you know is right for your child. With son #2, we insisted on testing in first grade, which led to early identification and early intervention. He did not fall as far behind and has progressed even beyond our first son. What you need to remember is that if you request testing, the school needs to do their evaluations first. You have to wait for the findings. If you disagree, you need to request a formal outside evaluation. The outside evaluation requires an appointment (sometimes with a wait as much as 6 six months), and then waiting for the results. The process takes time and the earlier you start the better. By the time son #1 finally began receiving special education services, the better part of the second grade was over. That's almost two whole academic years gone, when he should have been learning! Lastly, know that even if you are not sure of your decision, it is better than doing nothing. My husband always says: "Do something, even if it's wrong!" Doing nothing and waiting usually accomplishes exactly that – nothing. As a parent, trust your heart. My pediatrician told me early, that he always listens to what the mother says, because she can usually tell something is wrong long before even an expert specialist can, and is usually right! Reflect inwardly on how you feel; what you desire for your child, and then put your head down and move forward. Your child will ultimately be the one to benefit!

Mrs. Anderson: Surely the school would notice a remarkable improvement in behavior, once the child started medication, something that they cannot dismiss, and this change must be documented by the school in PPT minutes. If PPT was not scheduled, the mother must call an emergency PPT. By law, the school has five days to respond. Do not let the school say they have no more time for a PPT, because it is the end of the school year, and just shush the child off to summer school reading. At the PTT, the mother must come forward and disclose the facts that the child is under treatment for a psychiatric condition, and release the medication name (the nurse needs to know this anyway). This PPT now has a just cause for being called, as the mother has new information to add to the child's case. Upfront is the best approach for two reasons. First, it signals that the mom is proactive, and second, it alerts the school that there is a cause to put the child on the "watch-list", and they must now follow up with the same level of care the mother is providing from her end. As far as evaluations go – there is no just cause to provide psychological evaluation at this time. The only identified education related problem is reading. The next steps are to determine how far behind the child is in reading (insist on the low, median, and high levels in class to determine the lag), and to establish what the specific reason is for the child having reading problems. And this is where testing should be requested. There are several tests to determine the type of reading disorder and, based on the testing, there are different reading programs to teach reading, based on the child's specific reading problem. If the school can positively say, that the child could not learn to read because of the behavior issue, then they have a few weeks to determine if the child may respond to the summer reading program. If there is an improvement, then the child should go to summer school. If there is no improvement after two weeks, then the mother is to request one on one reading tutoring with the same number of hours as the school reading program. There is no time left before the summer break to perform reading testing, as they have something like forty five days to test and respond, plus another seven days to call a PPT. This is how the school can waste an entire year without doing anything for the child. The mother can request reading testing be performed over the summer with a PPT held within the first week of school to determine a reading plan. To send a child to a summer reading problem without identifying the cause of the problem is like treating a knee injury with shoulder physical therapy. It will cause additional problems in frustration and self-esteem, and may exasperate the preexisting mood issue. The mother should make this point at the PPT and insist, that any damage done from the lack of or an incorrect diagnosis at this point will cause regression. All of these key points are very important and must be documented in the meeting minutes.

The documentation is a key. There may not be a reason to label the child "special education" at this time, as reading problems can be corrected, and if the child is performing well under the supervision of the psychiatrist, then all is well. The mother should stay on top of this reading problem and require progress reports every three weeks to determine improvement. If there is no improvement, then the reading program should be changed. The most important educational statement I ever heard at a lecture was that children learn to read from K to 3rd grade, and then read to learn from then on. Any child who cannot read at 3rd grade has very little chance of ever catching up without serious intervention.

In the state of CA, they base the number of required prison cells by the number of children in the school system who cannot read by the third grade. If the school insists on using only one reading program that suits 95% of the population, then they have now made a stupid step (I kid you not: actual observance), and then it is time to get the big guns out with the assistance of an advocate. There is a very large possibility, that there may be additional mental health issues surfacing as the child gets older. If additional problems arise with mood and processing, then the mother should have the child labeled "special education" to assure the child's educational rights are protected under FAPE (free and public education act). The above are the first steps the mother must take at this time, no need to pull the cart before the donkey. I did hear of a report from a <u>noted</u> psychiatrist that was recently dismissed at a PPT. If I were that psychiatrist, I would be incensed by the lack of concern from the school administration. Over-document if necessary, vigilance is key. When a case goes to mediation, the only thing that hearing officer wants to see is documentation.

Recap
- Call Emergency PPT;
- Mother submits medical information;
- School to provide current reading level of child;
- School to provide reading levels of class;
- Mother to request testing for reading disorder;
- Mother to request a trial two week "summer reading program" to be introduced to child before year end;
- If improvement with reading, then child goes on to summer program;
- If no improvement then mother has to request one on one tutor; Mother to make all points at PPT;
- Mother to insure all points are documented in meeting minutes.

Note: the mother needs to take notes at the meeting and then compare to school issued minutes. If different, than the mother can submit an addendum to the minutes. The school must attach the addendum to the file. The best way is to hand deliver to the principal any documentations and letters.

Mrs. Hamilton: This lack of understanding and support hurts us, parents, and our children. There is a kid living in our block who has a brain tumor. He is quite debilitated and has a lot of attention. There are people coming to see him, fund raisers, meetings of support, balloons and such. My son is not less sick and debilitated than this kid, but he is avoided by his peers! Parents of other children do not want his company or play dates with him. We never saw a fund raiser or a meeting of support for children with mental illness and their parents, or balloons, or letters wishing my son to get well. It is sad and unfair. Our life is a constant battle to prove that our children are medically SICK, not spoiled or bad.

Dr.A: We all mentioned many times the importance of psychological testing. Diane Valentine, MS, ABSNP, CT Certified School Psychologist, Diplomate of American Board of School Neuropsychology, offered us her expert opinion on that matter.

Testing the Child with Disabilities

One of the most difficult tasks you face is to consign your child to the care and supervision of the local school district. For the parent of a child with a mental illness, the stakes are high. Trained to observe the signs that a child is on emotional overload, you can quickly assess a situation, and know what to do. You are the advocate, the expert; you represent your child's interests. Of course you want to protect your children against painful experiences. You may wonder, "Who will understand my child?" Since psychiatric illnesses are diagnosed through interview and observation, not through CT Scans or a blood test, a clinical symptom of your child's illness is often interpreted as a behavioral issue. You may spend a lot of time at school explaining, interpreting and intervening on behalf of your child.

It is common for children with emotional problems to have accompanying learning disabilities. Capable of competing with their classmates, at school they feel bewildered, befuddled and behind. They can't grasp concepts as quickly as others, and they don't know where to start when given assignments that require organization or planning. They forget lunch money, a pencil, permission slips signed, and their homework. Often, they decide they are not very smart so "who cares". Some quit trying, while others seek attention in negative ways. Social relationships suffer, behavior at school declines, and kids choose new and sometimes negative way to gain attention. This faulty reasoning can alter your child's future because he/she may stop trying to claim the rightful place at school and in life.

School failure is a painful experience for both parents and children, but can be avoided by carefully managing classroom placement, teacher selection, and available resources to support learning and emotional functioning. Your child may have learning difficulties, or behavioral problems, or both. It is important to find out what stands in the way of learning. Is it poor instruction; does your child have learning delays, or, a specific learning disability? Your child may be literally "unavailable", because learning can be "interrupted" by emotional problems or the side effects of medication. Often, the reasons for school problems are a combination of factors.

Although help in the classroom and learning accommodations can sometimes be informally arranged by talking to your child's teacher. Formal decisions about education are based on information obtained through various forms of intervention, testing, and through formal psychological testing. The purpose of formal testing is to determine whether your child has a significant problem in one of several areas related to the processing of information. These are called processing deficits, and they occur when testing shows, that your child has trouble interpreting information taken in through the senses.

The current federal definition specifies there must be a disorder in one or more of the basic psychological processes involved in understanding, or in using language, spoken or written, which may manifest itself in the imperfect ability to listen, think, speak, read, write, spell, or do mathematical calculations, including conditions such as perceptual disabilities, brain injury, minimal brain dysfunction, dyslexia, and developmental aphasia. (34 C.F.R. 300.7)

If your child has trouble copying from the board, reading quickly, or writing neatly and within margins, there might be a deficit in visual processing. Does your child seem to falter if given more than one direction at home, or have trouble remembering information at school presented orally? Does he/she have trouble with spelling or understanding what he/she reads? A school based psychological evaluation might identify a deficit in the way your child's brain recognizes and interprets sounds. Information from the evaluation will determine what remediation may be provided at school, as well as the level and intensity of services.

Psychological testing can provide an understanding of your child's learning style, including both strengths and weaknesses at a specific point in time. The testing will include an interview that establishes the reason for testing, a classroom observation, and instruments to assess intellectual functioning, behavior and personality. For test instruments, many schools use the Wechsler Scales, known as the WISC-IV, or the Woodcock-Johnson III Tests of Cognitive Abilities, known commonly as the WJ-III. Some test batteries include rating scales to measure behavior and emotional functioning. The rating scales are completed by parents, teachers, and your child. The finished "product", the psychological report, is reviewed at a formal meeting at school. Meeting participants include parents, classroom teachers, specialists such as the school psychologist, speech and language therapist, a representative from special education and an administrator. Results are discussed and decisions are made to benefit your child's learning needs. It's advisable to share the reports with members of your child's personal treatment team, including Pediatrician, Psychiatrist, Psychologist, or Counselor. The more professionals team with your family to benefit your child, the more success he/she would experience at home and school.

Psychological tests contain a selection of short subtests that measure specific skills needed for learning. For example, the Woodcock -Johnson "verbal comprehension" subtest is an oral test that has both a visual and an auditory component. It asks a child to identify objects from pictures, to name word opposites, and complete verbal analogies. It assesses verbal reasoning and language. Tests that require language synthesis using specific sounds may provide clues about the reasons your child has trouble reading.

Processing speed affects how the brain organizes information, and measures how quickly your child can scan and absorb information in order to read, write, and solve problems. As your child gets older and academic learning becomes more complex, the effects of a slow processing speed are significant. Here is an example: your child is watching television in the living room. He is told: "Put your backpack away, get dishes and silverware from the cupboard and set the table." If the child has trouble paying attention or remembering things he/she hears, the brain may be aware that someone said something, but what? The response in this case is: "huh?" Poor child! He/she hasn't processed the information. This same child may have trouble in the classroom when learning new information or making connections between the information seen on the page and what he/she already knows, because it is presented too quickly to hold in the memory. Slow processing can also damage social relations, as your child may have trouble visually interpreting social situations and making a quick, appropriate response.

Identifying the causes of slow processing requires true detective work, since there can be many explanations. For example, memory problems can slow down information processing. There may be problems in the way your child interprets what he/she sees or hears in the classroom. Emotional problems can interrupt and slow information processing, both with and without medication. Psychological testing can help sort it out.

Test scores are a source of anxiety for parents. What is a good score, and what score determines that there is a learning disability? Psychological test instruments are norm referenced. This means that the score is normed, or compared with a group of similar in age and other characteristics to your child. Your child's score is reported as a standard score.

While numbers are tantalizing to ponder, whether on a bathroom scale or on a final examination, they are not everything, when it comes to diagnosing a learning disability. Many years ago, schools made that diagnosis using a rigid mathematical algorithm called "Regression to the Mean". It described the statistical tendency for scores to average out. An average score on a test that measures intellectual functioning is 100, and about half the population score in the range of 90-110. Twenty five percent will be above the average range, and twenty five percent will be below the average range. In the curve you find the majority of scores. Today, schools are less rigid and evaluate your child's skills and the various skills needed to develop competency in reading, writing, and math. In fact, psychological, or norm-referenced testing, is often not the first choice, but the last choice after specific scientifically based interventions are completed.

Mrs. Anderson: I wish we could have this level of interaction and involvement of psychologists at schools! Finding right providers is as difficult and exhausting as climbing Mount Everest without equipment! What is going on with child psychiatrists? Are they becoming extinguished species? Especially the ones who are taking insurances? Are there any ways to find the "right" psychiatrist?

Dr. A: There are no simple or optimistic answers to those questions. To begin with, we are living in the time of health care crisis in general; mental health care getting the worst of it. Over the years we created a Frankenstein known as "managed care", although "mismanaged care" would be a more accurate description. It took years until we realized that managed care brought about the destruction of the health care system affecting every single person. Numerous armies of clerks find it possible to dictate to physicians how much time they should spend with every patient, what medications they are allowed to prescribe, and what procedures they can recommend. Essentially the treatment in all areas of medicine is defined by paper pushers, or medical doctors hired by insurances to find the reasons how not to recommend requested services, and how to spend the least amount of money possible on healthcare. In child psychiatry insurances approve what's called "medication management" for fifteen minutes. It turns out to be ten for the most part, between walking in and out of the office, writing prescriptions etc. For that length of time a psychiatrist is expected to talk to the child and the parent, discuss a treatment plan, side effects, progress at school, review different documentation. The interaction is not limited to the face to face visit: there are multiple calls from schools; communications with nurses, guidance counselors, psychologists and parents, when something does not go well, and the feedback is needed between appointments, filling out school forms, writing letters proving the need for special accommodations – to mention just a part of it. Most of the office visits are followed by about a double or triple amount of time spent on the phone or filling out the paperwork. And this is the time not recognized as "billable time" by insurances. Recently I learned that pediatricians started charging for filling out camp forms. They cannot be blamed for that: even five-ten minutes to spend on each form turn into huge amount of time, if multiplied by hundreds of kids leaving for camps every summer. Needless to say, that in a privately paid psychiatric office both children and their parents get more individual attention and time.

The first step toward choosing a psychiatrist is making a decision to use the insurance coverage, or a private pay doctor. A competent provider can be found under the insurance umbrella or outside it. Consider this: we pay money for a lot of services: hair cutting, plumbing, home improvement, vets, car services etc. Our health is crucial and more so our children's health. Paying for the treatment is a long term investment; parents are starting a relationship with a psychiatrist lasting for at least several years, and need to know that it is worth it. The search process became easier since all medical doctors have their credentials published on line as well as the feedback from their patients. But even with almighty Goggle the word of mouth remains the most reliable source of information. Parents of children with mental illness suffer from painful solitude and alienation until they find that there is a huge community of parents just like them, struggling with the same issues, ready to share their experience, finds and warnings. Some parents bring up at their visits cutting edge science questions, already discussed in the chat rooms, where the exchange of news flying back and forth is very intense. A local chat room becomes a valuable source of information: other parents would gladly recommend some psychiatrists and advise to avoid others. Still keep in mind that all recommendations are subjective – be they accolades or unflattering. There is a factor of individual compatibility, which defines the future success or failure of potential partnership. A controlling parent may feel uncomfortable with an assertive (and controlling) psychiatrist, who is a true expert and believes, that if a patient comes to see him/her, he is the one making decisions, and is not inclined to get into detailed discussions about the rational. On the other hand, a bewildered and perplexed parent might find it comforting and reassuring to work with the same psychiatrist, relying fully on the professional decisions and not agonizing about possible choices. These are just two opposite examples with many shades of grey in between. In other words, firstly parents are looking for a competent psychiatrist judged by his/her credentials as well as – possibly – feedback from the patients. Next comes a personal interview during which "the compatibility factor" needs to be looked at: the interaction between the child and the doctor (children and especially adolescent tend to open up more and participate in treatment, if they feel respected and heard), clarity of the explanations, ability to understand and address the problems in a compassionate way, and many other things, which fall under the nebulous umbrella of "chemistry". Yes, believe it or not, "chemistry" is important in child psychiatry; the sense of discomfort in the office might translate into noncompliance with treatment, and eventually into limited or no success. If you like and trust your psychiatrist and he/she is leaving the practice (Mrs. Hamilton case), or you are leaving the state consider asking for a referral to somebody he/she trusts. Sometimes the treatment is not progressing as well as everybody would hope, even with a "good" psychiatrist. In this case the question of a second opinion would come up, which is helpful for the parents as well as for the treating psychiatrist. Firstly ask him/her about the referral for the second opinion: if you trust your psychiatrist, this is the most reliable way to connect with the right person. A fresh eye may discover overlooked resources and help to move treatment forward. It is possible though that the second opinion would not add anything new, or would present with a totally opposite and even more confusing take on the treatment situation. In the latter case the parents need to make sure they understand why the second opinion is so drastically different and even write down the rational for this opinion, so it could be discussed with the "main" provider. Usually the need for the second opinion comes when children are going through puberty, and medications seem to stop working, or they develop unusual side effects on the majority of medications and need an "out of box" approach.

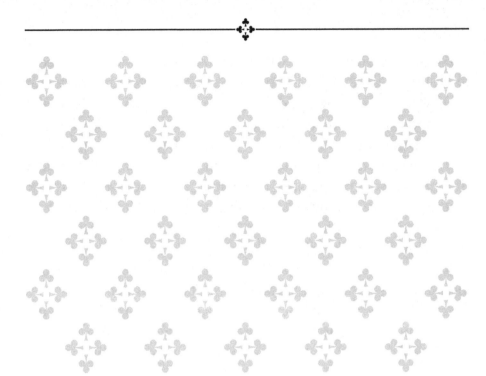

Epilogue
Will the House of Cards Hold?

Dear Reader, we are coming to the end of our story. Bringing up a child with mental illness is complex by itself, but the way our society views and treats mental health issues makes it even harder. Firstly we need to recognize that mental illness is as much of a medical condition as any other disease. It can start early with subtle prodromal symptoms, which should not be ignored, as we do not ignore difficulties in breathing, allergy and other medical conditions. Parents need to trust their judgment and seek help as soon as they notice any signs of abnormal development or behavior. Medical and educational systems are not prepared to deal adequately with mentally ill children: it takes a lot of determination and knowledge to get services children need. On the other hand, we know more now about the brain development and mental illness. We also have more medications in our psychiatric toolbox improving the quality of life and in some cases even eliminating symptoms of the disease. Parents have ways to get control over illness. Most importantly – you are not alone; there are many parents like you and more support than you can imagine.

As you can see - the house of cards holds!

Bibliography

J.T. Kantorowitz , D. C. Javitt. "Glutamate: new hope for schizophrenia treatment." Current Psychiatry, 2011; Vol. 10, No. 4, 69-71.

Elisabeth, Kubler – Ross. On Death and Dying. New York: Touchstone, 1969.

Sigmund, Freud. The Works of Sigmund Freud, 2010.

Emil Kraepelin. Manic- depressive Insanity and Paranoia, 2010.

Eugen Bleuler. Textbook of Psychiatry. MacMillan Co., 1924.

Charles Bradley, M. D. "The Behavior of Children Receiving Benzedrine." Am. J. Psychiatry, November 1937. No. 94, 577-585.

Leo Kanner. Childhood Psychosis: Initial Studies and New Insights. July 1, 1973.

Demitri, Papolos M.D. and Janice Papolos. The Bipolar Child. 2000

Thomas W. Phelan. 1-2-3 Magic: Effective Discipline for Children. 2012

Andrés Martin, Fred R. Volkmar and Melvin Lewis - Wolters. Lewis's Child and Adolescent Psychiatry: A Comprehensive Textbook. Kluwer Health/Lippincott Williams & Wilkins, 2007.

Wayne Hugo Green. Child and Adolescent Clinical Psychopharmacology (Green, Child and Adolescent Clinical Psychopharmacology). Lippincott 2006.

Andres Martin, Lawrence Scahill and Christopher Kratochvil. Pediatric Psychopharmacology. Oxford University Press, Inc., 2011.

Stephen M. Stahl. Stahl's Essential Psychopharmacology: Neuroscientific Basis and Practical Applications (Essential Psychopharmacology Series). Cambridge University Press, 2008.

Biederman J. and Spencer T. "Deficient emotional self-regulation and pediatric attention deficit hyperactivity disorder: a family risk analysis." Psychology Medicine, Aug 24, 2011: 1-8.

Liu HY, Potter MP, Woodworth KY, Yorks DM, Petty CR, Wozniak JR, Faraone SV and Biederman J. "Pharmacologic treatments for pediatric bipolar disorder: a review and meta-analysis." Journal of American Academic Child Adolescent Psychiatry. 2011 Aug; 50(8):749-62.e39.

Zukerman W. and Purcell A. Brain's synaptic pruning continues into your 20s. Pubmed, August 2011: 16:07 17.

Lewis S. "Development: Microglia go pruning, Nature Reviews." Neuroscience 12 September 2011: 492-493.

Paolicelli R. et al. Synaptic Pruning by Microglia Is Necessary for Normal Brain Development Published on line July 21,2011, Science DOI: 10.1126/science. 1202529

Hayashi-Takagi A. "Readdressing synaptic pruning theory for schizophrenia, Combination of brain imaging and cell biology" Commun Integr Biol. Mar-Apr 2011; 4(2): 211–212.

Shenton M. "A review of MRI findings in schizophrenia" Schizophrenia Research, 15 April 2001. Volume 49, Issue 1: 1-52.

Green J. "The SSRI Debate and the Evidence Base in Child and Adolescent Psychiatry" Curr Opin Psychiatry. 2004;17(4)

Fogel J, PhD. Stigma for Mental Disorders, Psychopharmacotherapeutic Drug Development, and Brief Dynamic Psychotherapy: Selected Sessions From the Canadian Academy of Child and Adolescent Psychiatry Meeting. March 2004.

White R., MD ; FRCPC and Giorgadze A., MD. "Child and Adolescent Psychiatry Viewpoint: Developmental Epidemiology" Journal of the American Academy of Child and Adolescent Psychiatry January 2006. Volume 45, Number 1: 8-25

White R., MD, FRCPC and Giorgadze A., MD. "Risperidone Maintenance for Disruptive Behavior Disorders" Am J Psychiatry. 2006; 163:402-410

White R., MD, FRCPC and Giorgadze A, MD. :Child and Adolescent Psychiatry Viewpoint: Old vs New Antipsychotics for EarlyOnset Schizophrenia." Eur Child Adolesc Psychiatry, 2006; Volume 14: 1-8.

Buck M. and Pharm.D., FCCP. "Escitalopram for the Treatment of Depression in Adolescents." Pediatr Pharm. 2009. 15(9).

Duffy A., Milin R. and Grof P. "Maintenance Treatment of Adolescent Bipolar Disorder: Open Study of the Effectiveness and Tolerability of Quetiapine." BMC Psychiatry. 2009; 9:4

Yellowlees P. MBBS, M.D. "Antidepressants and Childhood Suicidality: Are Fears Founded?" Medscape Psychiatry, October 2010.

West B. MPH. "Children at Risk for Suicide Attempt and Attempt-related Injuries: Findings from the 2007 Youth Risk Behavior Survey." Western J Emerg. Med. 2010; 11(3):257-263.

Hirst M., M.D. "Psychopharmacology for Children With Advanced Illnesses a Challenge." Medscape Psychiatry. March 2011.

Culpepper L., M.D., MPH. "Recognizing Suicide Risk Factors in Primary and Psychiatric Care." Medscape Psychiatry. October 2010.

Compton M., M.D., MPH. "Children of Parents With Mental Illnesses: When to Intervene." Medscape Psychiatry. August 2011.

Compton M., MD, MPH. "A Look at Mental Health and the Court System." Medscape Psychiatry. August 2011.

Curry J., Silva S. and Rohde P. "Recovery and recurrence following treatment for adolescent major depression." Arch Gen Psychiatry. 2011; 68:263–9.

O'Shaughnessy R. M.D. "Forensic Psychiatry and Violent Adolescents." Brief Treat Crisis Interv. 2008;8(1):27-42.

Soh N. "Walter G. Complementary Medicine for Psychiatric Disorders in Children and Adolescents." Curr Opin Psychiatry. 2008;21(4):350-355.

Hunt K. and Coelh H. "Complementary and Alternative Medicine Use in England: Results from a National Survey" Int. J. Clin. Pract. 2010; 64(11):1496-1502.

Woodard R. "The Diagnosis and Medical Treatment of ADHD in Children and Adolescents in Primary Care: A Practical Guide." Pediatr Nurs. 2006; 32(4):363-370.

Sharp S. and Hellings J. "Efficacy and Safety of Selective Serotonin Reuptake Inhibitors in the Treatment of Depression in Children and Adolescents." Clin. Drug Invest. 2006; 26(5):247-255.

Brent D. "Early Interventions May Lower Risks for Suicide Reattempts in Adolescents." J Am Acad Child Adolesc Psychiatry. 2009;48:977–978, 987–996, 997–1004, 1005–1013

Côté S.M. "Depression and Anxiety Symptoms: Onset, Developmental Course and Risk Factors During Early Childhood." J Child Psychol Psychiatry. 2009 Oct; 50(10):1201-8.

Piacentini J. and Woods D.W. "Behavior Therapy for Children with Tourette's Disorder: A Randomized Controlled Trial. JAMA. May 19, 2010. 303(19):1929-37. Jankovic J. "Tourette's syndrome." N Engl J Med. Oct 18 2001; 345(16):1184-92. Medline.

Bohlhalter S. "Neural Correlates of Tic Generation in Tourette's Syndrome: An Event-related Functional MRI Study." Brain. Aug 2006;129:2029-37. Medline

Singer H.S. "Tourette's Syndrome: From Behavior to Biology." Lancet Neurol. Mar 2005;4(3):149-59. Medline

Ross RG. "New Findings on Antipsychotic Use in Children and Adolescents with Schizophrenia Spectrum Disorders." Am J Psychiatry. November 2008. 165(11):1369-72.

Asarnow R.F. "Schizophrenia and Schizophrenia-spectrum Personality Disorders in the First-Degree Relatives of Children with Schizophrenia: The UCLA Family Study." Arch Gen Psychiatry Jun 2001;58(6):581-8. Medline.

Keshavan M.S. "Premorbid Characterization in Schizophrenia: The Pittsburgh High Risk Study." World Psychiatry. October 2004. 3(3):163-8. Medline.

Gogtay N. "Structural Brain MRI Abnormalities in Healthy Siblings of Patients with Childhood-onset Schizophrenia. Am J Psychiatry. March 2003. 160(3):569-71. Medline

Weinberger D.R. and McClure R.K. "Neurotoxicity, Neuroplasticity, and Magnetic Resonance Imaging Morphometry: What is Happening in the Schizophrenic Brain?." Arch Gen Psychiatry. Jun 2002;59(6):553-8. Medline

Rapoport J.L. "Progressive Cortical Change During Adolescence in Childhood-onset Schizophrenia. A Longitudinal Magnetic Resonance Imaging Study." Arch Gen Psychiatry. July 1999. 56(7):649-54. Medline.

Rapoport J.L. "The Neurodevelopmental Model of Schizophrenia: Update 2005." Mol Psychiatry. May 2005; 10(5):434-49. Medline.

Holi M,M, "Detecting Suicidality Among Adolescent Outpatients: Evaluation of Trained Clinicians' Suicidality Assessment Against a Structured Diagnostic Assessment Made by Trained Raters." BMC Psychiatry. December 31, 2008. 8: 97.

Luby J.L. "Preschool Depression: Homotypic Continuity and Course Over 24 Months." Arch Gen Psychiatry. August 2009. 66(8):897-905.